SEX
and Diabetes

For Him and For Her

Janis Roszler, RD, CDE, LDN & Donna Rice, MBA, BSN, RN, CDE
FOREWORD BY JOYCELYN ELDERS, MD

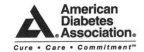

American
Diabetes
Association®
Cure • Care • Commitment™

Director, Book Publishing, Rob Anthony; *Managing Editor*, Abe Ogden; *Editor*, Rebekah Renshaw; *Production Manager*, Melissa Sprott; *Composition*, ADA; *Cover Design*, ADA; *Printer:* Victor Graphics, Inc.

Printed in the United States of America
1 3 5 7 9 10 8 6 4 2

The suggestions and information contained in this publication are generally consistent with the *Clinical Practice Recommendations* and other policies of the American Diabetes Association, but they do not represent the policy or position of the Association or any of its boards or committees. Reasonable steps have been taken to ensure the accuracy of the information presented. However, the American Diabetes Association cannot ensure the safety or efficacy of any product or service described in this publication. Individuals are advised to consult a physician or other appropriate health care professional before undertaking any diet or exercise program or taking any medication referred to in this publication. Professionals must use and apply their own professional judgment, experience, and training and should not rely solely on the information contained in this publication before prescribing any diet, exercise, or medication. The American Diabetes Association—its officers, directors, employees, volunteers, and members—assumes no responsibility or liability for personal or other injury, loss, or damage that may result from the suggestions or information in this publication.

♾ The paper in this publication meets the requirements of the ANSI Standard Z39.48-1992 (permanence of paper).

ADA titles may be purchased for business or promotional use or for special sales. For information, please write to: Lee Romano Sequeira, Special Sales & Promotions, at the address below, or at LRomano@diabetes.org or 703-299-2046.
For all other inquiries, please call 1-800-DIABETES.

American Diabetes Association
1701 North Beauregard Street
Alexandria, Virginia 22311

Library of Congress Cataloging-in-Publication Data
Roszler, Janis.
  Sex and diabetes : for him and for her / Janis Roszler and Donna Rice.
     p. cm.
  Includes index.
  ISBN 978-1-58040-277-4 (alk. paper)
  1. Diabetics—Sexual behavior. 2. Diabetes—Complications. I. Rice, Donna (Donna M.) II. Title.
RC660.4.R6892 2007
616.4'62—dc22

2007018996

To my terrific sisters, Lisa and Elaine
—Janis

To my mother, Christine,
and my wonderful sons, David and Douglas
—Donna

Contents

Acknowledgments. vii

Foreword ix

Chapter 1 The Passion in Your Life 1

Chapter 2 Diabetes and Your Feelings. . . 13

Chapter 3 Diabetes and Your Body 33

Chapter 4 For Him. 53

Chapter 5 For Her 71

Chapter 6 For Fun 89

Chapter 7 For Couples. 111

Chapter 8 Don't Try This at Home 123

Chapter 9 As We Age 135

Chapter 10 Speaking with Your Doctor. . . 153

Chapter 11 Recipes for Love 163

Chapter 12 Resources. 181

Appendix. 189

Index 197

Acknowledgments

I would like to thank:

Botsford Hospital in Farmington Hills, Michigan, for having the vision and insight to serve the educational needs of the community and to support a program that touches so many lives.

Steven J. Roth, DO, for his guidance, mentorship, and endless support to help launch such a worthwhile program focusing on the sexuality needs of people with chronic illnesses.

I would especially like to thank the many men and women with diabetes, who have contributed to my knowledge and expertise by providing me the opportunity to help them overcome this very devastating complication. You are truly my teachers!

—Donna Rice

I would like to thank:

Maxine Cohn and Lisa Bauch for their editing expertise. Dr. Justin Grady Matrisciano, founder of *www.cartoonmd.com*, for his artistic talent. Landi Turner for her wisdom and enthusiasm.

The fabulous gang at www.dLife.com. All the contributors willing to share their heartfelt stories on the www.dearjanis.com message boards.

Robert Anthony of the American Diabetes Association for inviting us to bring this important topic to print.

—Janis Roszler

Foreword

How exciting! When I received the invitation to write the foreword to *Sex and Diabetes*, I immediately became quite nostalgic. As Surgeon General of the United States (1993-1994) during the Clinton administration, I voiced the need for a responsible and comprehensive sex education program for our nation, and now, to my great delight, I have the opportunity to speak again about this very topic.

Humans are passionate beings who love to be loved, held, and connected to others on both a physical and emotional level. This closeness affects our quality of life and ability to withstand the stresses of an ever-changing world. Our intimate relationships support us through tough times and also help us celebrate joyous ones.

When these intimate bonds are hampered by a medical condition like diabetes, the negative effects can resonate throughout every area of our lives—our support systems can become strained, our self-confidence may wane, and our ability to face daily health challenges can waver. Sadly, as important as this area of our life is to our overall health, very few people with sexual complications seek help and only a handful of medical professionals will mention this topic during a visit.

This book is long overdue. As one of the first books on diabetes-related sexual complications, I am certain that it will help a great number of individuals. *Sex and Diabetes* discusses diabetes-related sexual complications in both men and women, offers treatment options, suggests ways to enhance intimate communication, teaches how to avoid fraudulent products, offers advice on how to discuss sexual complications with a health care provider, and even suggests ways to help rekindle the romance and fun in your relationship. It even contains a delicious assortment of enticing aphrodisiac recipes!

Enjoy this book. Use it to help guide you to a more fulfilling and meaningful intimate relationship. Share it with someone you love and use that strength to enrich all areas of your life.

Joycelyn Elders, MD
Former Surgeon General of the United States (1993-1994)
Distinguished Professor of Public Health
University of Arkansas Medical School

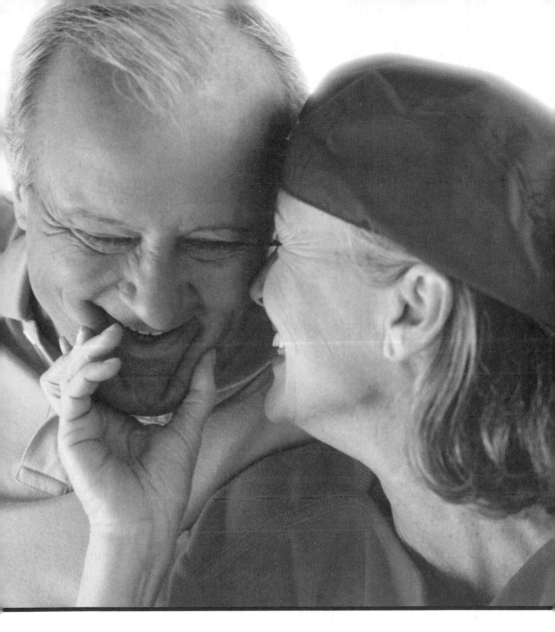

Chapter 1
The Passion in Your Life

In this chapter:
▌ Examine two different types of intimacy.
▌ Identify intimacy problems that may develop with diabetes.

WOULD THE LOVE of an amazing woman motivate you to build a monument that would be visited by millions? Could the passion that you feel for an incredible man drive you to conquer countries? Great loves have existed from the beginning of time and still exist today. Since the time of Adam and Eve, men and women have connected sexually with one another, and these relationships have created some of the most romantic and exciting stories ever told. The stories retold throughout this chapter are a testament to the power and intensity of the human connection.

THE TWO TYPES OF INTIMACY

Two types of intimacy, physical and emotional, played an enormous role in the lives of some of history's greatest loves. They can be part of our lives as well.

Physical intimacy

Physical intimacy is all about touch. It involves holding, caressing, sexual attraction, and intimate actions. It is the subject of love songs, poems, and romantic stories. Physical intimacy is what many of us yearn for when we are alone and is what we feel when we connect with someone in a romantic way.

We not only crave the touch of another human being because of the potential pleasure that it brings; the touch of others can help us survive. Research studies show that newborns need a loving touch to develop normally. Within the first few days after birth, infants who are held in their mothers' loving arms maintain a healthier body temperature than those who are left alone. Young children who are not held or hugged may be at a greater risk for developing body image problems, such as anorexia or bulimia, as they grow. And this need for physical intimacy does not diminish with time. In our golden years, the desire to be sexually active rarely wanes, as many seniors report that they still feel a deep longing for a sexual relationship that includes touching and kissing.

Emotional intimacy

Emotional intimacy is what happens inside of our heads. It is the non-physical sharing of two people who care deeply about one another. You

HISTORIC ROMANCES:
Cleopatra and Marc Antony

Cleopatra VII, one of the most famous rulers of Egypt, lived a life that was filled with deep and intense sexual activity. As demanded by her position, she initially married her younger brother, Ptolemy, but later became the mistress of the Roman general Julius Caesar. Following Caesar's death, she discovered her true love— Marc Antony, who had arrived in Egypt to expand the ever-growing Roman Empire. Their affair was scandalous. Despite the protests and risks involved, Marc Antony and Cleopatra married in 36 B.C. and plotted to conquer Rome and claim it as their own. But tragedy struck. Antony heard a false report that Cleopatra had died and fell upon his own sword to end his life. With her beloved Antony dead, Cleopatra took her life by coaxing a poisonous asp to bite her.

have emotional intimacy with another person when you feel confident that he or she accepts you for who you are. It develops when you and someone you love share experiences together. You know how your partner wants a morning cup of coffee and can anticipate how she will react to a situation before it happens. It is this bond that takes your partnership to a higher level.

Many experts suggest that the brain is the sexiest organ of all. When an emotional connection develops between two individuals that is built on mutual respect and caring, the relationship becomes far more precious. Physical intimacy is enjoyable on its own, but when combined with emotional intimacy, the passion that develops is special indeed.

THE HUMAN REACTION

When we fall in love, two chemicals are released—phenyethylamine (PEA) and norepinephrine. PEA is an amphetamine-like substance that elevates our moods and helps create the feeling of falling in love that so many of us enjoy. One reason chocolate is such a sought-after delight is because it is a source of PEA. When we eat it, we experience a feeling that

HISTORIC ROMANCES:
Shah Jahan and Arjumand Banu Begum

India's stunningly beautiful Taj Mahal was built as a monument to memorialize the love that Emperor Shah Jahan had for his wife. Shah Jahan was born in 1592. At the young age of 14, he met Arjumand Banu Begum, the prime minister's 15-year-old daughter and was immediately smitten. He quickly ran off to purchase a diamond for the price of 10,000 rupees ($300) and announced his desire to take her as his wife. The couple married five years later. When he ascended to the throne in 1628, he included his wife in many legislative duties and she accompanied him on military campaigns and even advised him on affairs of state. He adored her and called her Mumtaz Mahal, the "jewel of the palace." She was loved and admired by her people, was famous for her generosity, and was considered a woman of legendary beauty and virtue.

But tragedy entered the lives of the two lovers when Mumtaz Mahal died while giving birth to their 14th child. Shah Jahan was heartbroken. Determined to find a way to keep her memory alive, he emptied most of the money from the royal treasury and fulfilled his wife's dying wish—he built a monument, the famous Taj Mahal, to memorialize their love. Eventually, Shah Jahan fell ill and a struggle for the throne began. Shah Jahan's son, Aurangzeb, imprisoned him and kept him from his most precious possession—his view of the Taj Mahal. Fortunately, he was able to procure a tiny mirror, which caught the reflection of his treasured building and enabled him to see it once again. When he died in 1666, he was buried in the Taj Mahal with his wife.

resembles this warm and wonderful emotion. Similarly, norepinephrine has the following effects:

- elevates our blood pressure
- raises heart rate
- causes our palms to sweat
- forms an intense connection to the object of our attraction

Think back to your first love. If you became tongue-tied, sweaty, and nervous, you felt this way because of the norepinephrine in your system.

When Cupid's arrow strikes and these chemicals are released, our bodies respond more intensely, especially if we are able to transform our attraction into a physical relationship.

When a man experiences a stimulating touch, smell, vision, or thought, his brain activates a group of nerves that tell the tissues of the penis to relax. This allows blood to flow into two tubes inside of the penis that are known as corpora cavernosa. As they fill up, they press onto the veins that usually allow blood to exit and prevent fluid from escaping. The penis then becomes erect and prepares the body for intimacy with a partner. Stimulation causes the penis to contract and send semen out through the urethra, the tube that normally carries urine out from the body. The pleasurable sensation that is felt when this occurs is called an orgasm.

A woman's response to sexual stimulation is usually more subtle. Unlike a man, whose reaction is almost immediate, a woman's arousal is on a slow "simmer" that gradually increases in intensity. To fully enjoy the sexual experience, most women must connect both mentally and physically with their partner. The more emotionally involved a woman is with her partner, the more enthusiastically her body will often respond. As her state of arousal heightens, her breathing, heart rate, and blood pressure increase. Blood accumulates in various regions of her body, causing her skin to flush. The vaginal area swells and lubricates in anticipation of sexual intercourse and tension develops throughout her body until an orgasm occurs. When all parts of one's body are functioning as they should, the sexual act can be fulfilling and raise a relationship to a higher level.

Physical and emotional connections do more than inspire great nations to be conquered, buildings to be built, and poetry to be composed,

> When an emotional connection develops between two individuals that is built on mutual respect and caring, the relationship becomes far more precious.

they bind two people together in a way that can withstand any physical or emotional challenge. When diabetes enters your relationship, however, it can affect how you relate to your partner on both a physical and emotional level.

You may not be ready to erect massive monuments, fall onto a sword, or compose poetry that will be quoted by generations to come, but the intimate relationship that you have with a loved one deserves to be cherished, nurtured, and protected. Remember how you fell in love? What it was like to be together intimately for the first time? How about the wonderful "pillow talk" that you enjoyed after sharing an intimate embrace? If diabetes has stolen romance from your relationship, you can bring it back. Don't deny yourself the most intimate expression of caring that a couple can share.

This book should be able to provide you with guidance. Diabetes may change the way you experience certain pleasurable moments in your life, but it doesn't have to steal them from you altogether. You can enjoy a new level of intimacy with your partner. As the comedian Joan Rivers likes to ask, "Can we talk?" Yes we can.

FOR YOU AND YOUR PARTNER

1 Answer the quizzes found at the end of this chapter (pp. 8–11).

2 Discuss your results with each other and identify issues of concern and misunderstanding.

3 Keep these issues in mind as you read this book.

HISTORIC ROMANCES:

Robert Browning and Elizabeth Barrett

More than 500 heartfelt letters were exchanged between poets Robert Browning and Elizabeth Barrett. When they first met, Elizabeth was a recluse, having suffered for years with a lung ailment and, later in life, a spinal injury resulting from a horse riding accident. She was also deeply depressed after the tragic drowning death of her brother. But in 1844, Robert sought her out after admiring her poems and brought her back to life. They were determined to be together forever. Elizabeth's father bitterly opposed the romance, so the couple secretly married in 1846 and ran off to live in Florence, Italy. There, her health improved and she gave birth to a son. Elizabeth died on June 29, 1861. Their love was forever memorialized in verse:

"Sonnets from the Portuguese 43"

"How do I love thee…"
by Elizabeth Barrett Browning (1806–1861)

How do I love thee? Let me count the ways.
I love thee to the depth and breadth and height
My soul can reach, when feeling out of sight
For the ends of Being and ideal Grace.
I love thee to the level of everyday's
Most quiet need, by sun and candlelight.
I love thee freely, as men strive for Right;
I love thee purely, as they turn from Praise.
I love thee with a passion put to use
In my old griefs, and with my childhood's faith.
I love thee with a love I seemed to lose
With my lost saints, —I love thee with the breath,
Smiles, tears, of all my life! —and, if God choose,
I shall but love thee better after death.

QUIZ 1:
Have Diabetes-Related Sexual Complications Entered Your Life? (for men)

1. Have you been experiencing difficulty recently in achieving erections that you and your partner consider adequate for vaginal intercourse?
   ☐ Yes ☐ No

2. Do you have difficulty performing intercourse in more than half of your attempts?
   ☐ Yes ☐ No

3. Does this problem with erection difficulty occur when you are with a partner?
   ☐ Yes ☐ No

4. Does this problem with erection difficulty occur when you are alone?
   ☐ Yes ☐ No

5. How often have you been experiencing difficulty in achieving erections?
   ☐ Never ☐ Sometimes ☐ Most times ☐ Always

6. Does it take longer to achieve an erection than in the past?
   ☐ Yes ☐ No

7. Has it become more difficult to have intercourse in certain positions?
   ☐ Yes ☐ No

8. Have you ever been told that you have some form of cardiovascular disease or heart disease?
   ☐ Yes ☐ No

9. Have you ever been told that you have an elevated cholesterol level?
   ☐ Yes ☐ No

10. Has your desire for intercourse changed?
    ☐ Yes ☐ No

11. Has your partner's desire for intercourse changed?
☐ Yes ☐ No

12. Is your blood sugar under control?
☐ Never ☐ Sometimes ☐ Most times ☐ Always

13. Do you know your average blood sugar level (A1C)?
☐ Yes ☐ No

14. Have you ever checked your blood sugar level before or after sexual intercourse?
☐ Yes ☐ No

15. If yes, do you experience hypoglycemia (low blood sugar) with this activity?
☐ Yes ☐ No

16. Do you feel that diabetes is a cause of your sexual problem?
☐ Yes ☐ No

17. Has your sexual problem interfered with your relationship with your partner?
☐ Yes ☐ No

18. Has your sexual problem interfered with your job?
☐ Yes ☐ No

19. Has your sexual problem interfered with your family?
☐ Yes ☐ No

20. Are you feeling depressed over this problem?
☐ Yes ☐ No

QUIZ 2:
Have Diabetes-Related Sexual Complications Entered Your Life? (for women)

1. Describe your desire for intercourse.
   ☐ Poor   ☐ Fair   ☐ Strong   ☐ Very Strong

2. Describe your partner's desire for intercourse.
   ☐ Poor   ☐ Fair   ☐ Strong   ☐ Very Strong

3. Are you able to reach orgasm with intercourse?
   ☐ Never   ☐ Sometimes   ☐ Most times   ☐ Always

4. Are you able to reach orgasm when you are alone?
   ☐ Never   ☐ Sometimes   ☐ Most times   ☐ Always

5. Do you have a decreased amount of vaginal lubrication?
   ☐ Never   ☐ Sometimes   ☐ Most times   ☐ Always

6. Is your blood sugar under control?
   ☐ Never   ☐ Sometimes   ☐ Most times   ☐ Always

7. Do you know your average blood sugar level (A1C)?
   ☐ Yes   ☐ No

8. Have you checked your blood sugar before or after sexual intercourse?
   ☐ Yes   ☐ No

9. If yes, do you experience hypoglycemia (low blood sugar) with this activity?
   ☐ Yes   ☐ No

10. Do you have frequent vaginal and/or bladder infections?
    ☐ Yes   ☐ No

11. Is intercourse painful?
    ☐ Yes   ☐ No

12. Has your sexual problem interfered with your relationship with your partner?
    ☐ Yes   ☐ No

13. Has your sexual problem interfered with your job?
    ☐ Yes   ☐ No

14. Has your sexual problem interfered with your family?
    ☐ Yes   ☐ No

15. Are you feeling very depressed over this problem?
    ☐ Yes   ☐ No

You've just completed an important pretest. If any of the comments that you responded to indicate the presence of a problem or highlight an issue that you would like to learn more about, read on.

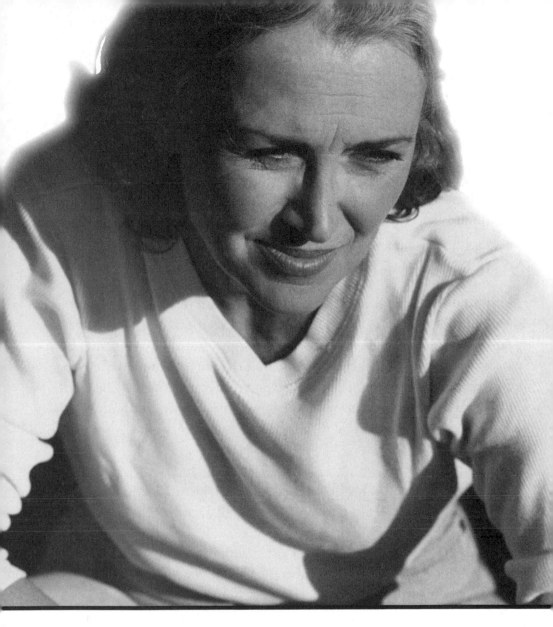

Chapter 2
Diabetes and Your Feelings

In this chapter:
▮ Explore some of the feelings that you may have with diabetes.
▮ Learn different ways to deal with them.

IF YOU HAVE DIABETES, it can affect the emotional and physical aspects of your intimate relationship. Let's first discuss the emotional concerns.

Diabetes is never welcomed with open arms. It frequently stirs up difficult emotions, including fear and guilt. If permitted to thrive, these emotions can create a rift in your relationship and cause you to lose one of the most important supporters in your effort to lead a healthy and meaningful life.

YOU MAY FEEL GUILTY

Many emotions arise when you are diagnosed with diabetes, but guilt should not be one of them. You may feel that your diabetes magically appeared because of something that you did or ate, but that is not true. Each person who develops diabetes has inherited the potential to have it. We know that there is no way to prevent type 1, and type 2 has several environmental triggers—such as weight gain and inactivity—but both types require an inherited potential for the disease to develop.

Risk factors

There are certain risk factors that experts have identified that make a person more susceptible to developing type 2 diabetes:

- If you are 45 years old or older
- If you have a parent, brother, or sister with diabetes
- If you have had gestational diabetes (diabetes during pregnancy) or have given birth to a baby that weighed more than 9 pounds
- If you are of African-American, Latino, Native-American, Asian-American, or Pacific-Islander descent
- If you were diagnosed with prediabetes
- If you have polycystic ovarian syndrome (PCOS)

Think of all of the people you know who are overweight and inactive and don't have diabetes; not everyone develops it. What you eat, how you behave, and health decisions that you have made over the years are not the sole cause of your disease, so don't permit overwhelming feelings of guilt to place a wedge between you and the people you love.

Impact of Guilt on Marriage

"Because of my type 2 diabetes, Julie and I can't be spontaneous anymore. Before we go out for the evening, we must plan everything around my eating schedule. If my blood sugar goes low, we can't leave until I feel better. If my headache remains after treating my low, we'll often cancel our plans altogether. How can she enjoy this? I sure don't. If I had eaten less and exercised more, I wouldn't have diabetes right now. My family says that I did this to myself and I believe them. If I didn't have diabetes, Julie and I could enjoy more activities together. Instead, I've ruined our lives. She should be with someone else." —*Rick*

Your partner may share your feelings of guilt, especially if he or she supported your desire to bring junk food into the house or watch television instead of heading out for a walk or exercise class. These feelings can bring a great deal of tension into the home. To help deal with any guilty feelings that either of you may have, learn as much as you can about diabetes and incorporate new health behaviors in your home. The changes that you make are healthy for the entire family.

The positive side of diabetes

Surprisingly, many people feel thankful that diabetes is now part of their lives. Before their diagnosis, they were sedentary, made poor food choices, their weight was significantly higher than it should have been, and they felt sluggish and unmotivated. Once diabetes came on the scene, they initially felt overwhelming feelings of guilt and so did their partner. But those feelings passed quickly as soon as they began to take control of their diabetes.

Open up about your feelings

The more that you and your partner know about this disease and what you can do to attain better control and reduce your risk of complications, the more comfortable you should both feel about the future that you can share together. Discuss your concerns with your partner. If you suspect that he or she feels negatively about your diabetes, talk about it. You may

Turning Your Life Around

"I used to be the fat guy that you would stare at in the grocery store. My cart would be filled with high-fat desserts, sausages, regular soda, chips, and more. When diabetes hit, I immediately felt that I had done it to myself. In the back of my mind, I knew that it would happen and then one day it did. Wham! When I got that blood test report back from the doctor, I felt my stomach sink. All I could think was, 'why didn't I say no to the choices I made?' When my wife learned about my diabetes, she immediately blamed herself. For years, she supported all of the bad behaviors that I had developed. We both ordered in pizza and drank beer on Saturday nights. We both sat in front of the television for hours on end snacking on junk food and sugary sodas. And we both never made a move to … move! We didn't do any physical activity of any type. Suddenly, the diabetes that I had caused was going to ruin both of our lives and our dream of us growing old together.

Fortunately, my doctor insisted that we attend the diabetes classes at the local hospital. I learned how to make better food choices, checked my blood sugar regularly, began walking each day, and started to lose some weight. Lucy joined me for the walks, which made them far more enjoyable. I began to feel younger than I had felt in a very long time. I was becoming healthier and more energetic. If I hadn't been diagnosed with diabetes, I never would have made any of these changes. Now I'm in far better shape than many of my friends. It sounds strange to thank diabetes for anything, but I really do. And so does my wife. With my previous lifestyle, she always believed that she would end up as a young widow. Now that I've changed so dramatically, we both look forward to a bright future together." —*Chuck*

be right about your partner's feelings or you may discover that this is not how he or she feels at all. An honest and open discussion will hopefully provide you with information that you can use to help strengthen your relationship.

YOU MAY FEEL DEPRESSED

About 30% of all individuals with diabetes experience some form of depression. Why these two conditions tend to go hand in hand is not clearly understood, but we do know that having diabetes doubles the risk of becoming depressed. When you are depressed, you may experience:

∎ a loss of interest in things that you used to enjoy
∎ guilt
∎ a sense of worthlessness
∎ a drop in your energy level
∎ too much or too little sleep
∎ withdrawal from friends and family
∎ physical pain
∎ loss of desire or physical ability to connect intimately with the one you love

Feelings of depression can be overwhelming and affect every area of your life, including your intimate relationship. Individuals with depression describe how they feel in a variety of different ways. Some say that they feel blue or numb, while others experience actual physical aches and pain.

Depression's Toll on Marriage

Mark has had type 2 diabetes for several years. He never paid much attention to it, because he always felt fine. Recently, however, Mark and his family have noticed a very definite change in his behavior and attitude toward the things that he used to enjoy. He no longer asks his wife and children about their day when he arrives home from the office. He doesn't plan family activities for the weekends like he used to do. All he does is lie down on the couch and watch television. He doesn't even care what's on. He'll watch old movies, reality shows, and even the poorly written sitcoms that he always considered to be a waste of time. Nowadays, he feels so tired that he can't muster up enough energy to do much else. At first, his wife worried that he was ill, but that concern quickly turned into frustration. He never listens to her, doesn't compliment her on anything she does, and no longer wants to join her for a night out to see a movie or be with friends. Mark is depressed and it is affecting their relationship.

Physical Effects of Depression

"I have had type 1 diabetes for about eight years. I used to have so much joy in my day. Tom and I loved holding hands as we watched television. The little things made us happy. Now I can barely get out of bed. Don't even mention romance to me. I don't want any part of it. I feel like I have a flu that won't leave." — *Diane*

Coping with depression

Depression can be challenging to deal with, but there are several things you can do to help improve your situation.

Depression Risk Assessment

Take the following assessment exercise to see if your feelings of depression require more urgent medical attention. Circle the number for each statement that best describes how often you felt or behaved this way during the past week.

Feelings	Rarely (less than 1 day)	Occasionally or a little of the time (1–2 days)	Some of the time (3–4 days)	All of the time (5–7 days)
I was bothered by things that don't usually bother me.	0	1	2	3
I did not feel like eating, my appetite was poor.	0	1	2	3
I felt that I could not shake off the blues even with help from my family or friends.	0	1	2	3
I felt that I was just as good as other people.	3	2	1	0
I had trouble keeping my mind on what I was doing.	0	1	2	3
I felt depressed.	0	1	2	3
I felt that everything I did was an effort.	0	1	2	3
I felt hopeful about the future.	3	2	1	0

Keep your blood sugar level in a healthy range

High and low glucose levels can cause emotional swings and exhaust you. Your partner may find your mood swings challenging as well. It is more difficult to connect romantically with someone whose demeanor can't be predicted. Ways to accomplish this goal will be discussed in greater detail in chapter 3.

Participate in some form of physical activity every day

Exercise releases endorphins ("happy hormones") that lift your spirit and help fight mild depression. Sexual activity is a healthy form of exercise also. Don't underestimate the mental and physical value of connecting with a person in an intimate way.

I thought my life had been a failure.	0	1	2	3
I felt fearful.	0	1	2	3
My sleep was restless.	0	1	2	3
I was happy.	3	2	1	0
I talked less than usual.	0	1	2	3
I felt lonely.	0	1	2	3
I felt people were unfriendly.	0	1	2	3
I enjoyed life.	3	2	1	0
I had crying spells.	0	1	2	3
I felt sad.	0	1	2	3
I felt that people disliked me.	0	1	2	3
I could not get going.	0	1	2	3

Adapted from page 185 of *Diabetes Burnout*, by William H. Polonsky, PhD, CDE, American Diabetes Association, 1999.

Scoring the Depression Risk Assessment

To determine your score, add up your responses to all of the questions: _____

If your total score is 16 or higher, you should consider taking action immediately—contact your health professional for a referral to a qualified mental health professional.

If you feel depressed, but your score is below 16, don't ignore your feelings. You can still speak with your health care team about how you feel.

Share your problems with a qualified counselor

It can be helpful to talk over your relationship problems with a neutral third party. Ask a member of your health care team for a referral.

Discuss your feelings with your physician

There are many different depression medications available today that are quite effective. One may work for you.

Pray or connect with your church, synagogue, or spiritual group

Research shows that people who have a spiritual connection handle the challenges of diabetes better than those who don't.

The emotional connection that you create with your partner is important for your relationship. If that area of your life has been altered because of your diabetes, do what you can to heal it. It will help you enjoy the intimate life that you want and deserve.

YOU MAY FEEL STRESSED

The stress of living with any disease can affect your energy level, how you feel about yourself, and how you relate to your partner. Life with a chronic disease like diabetes can be exhausting. When you live with diabetes, you must focus on a number of factors at once. A few of these factors are:

- food choices
- medication
- physical activity
- blood glucose testing
- foot care

In order to have good diabetes control, you must monitor your life closely. If you are emotionally and physically exhausted from the tasks that you need to do each day to maintain your health, you will have less to offer your loved one. Bedtime will become a time to collapse and fall asleep. When you add other responsibilities to the mix, such as children, homework, carpool, elderly parents, shopping, cleaning, and working, it's no surprise that you have little energy left to participate fully in the bedroom.

Exhaustion From Daily Diabetes Maintenance

"I hate sticking my fingers. I think about it most of the day. I test before meals to provide my doctor with the information that he wants and then test two hours after my meals so I can check if I balanced my insulin and food intake well. I check my feet each night and brush and floss my teeth so I don't develop any oral infections. When I shop, I read labels to check out the carbohydrate content of the foods that I purchase. I watch the clock to make certain that I don't miss a feeding or dose of medicine. Frankly, I'm pooped! After all of this, I can't gather up any additional energy to go home from work and be a fabulous partner in the bedroom. When my head hits the pillow, I'm out for the night."—*Kim*

Reducing your stress level

Here are some steps that you can take to help reduce your stress level:

Adjust your job duties

If your workload is overwhelming, try to share some of the load with a coworker. If your current position is too stressful, consider switching to a different one or see if the duties of the job can be altered in some way. You may feel additional stress if you don't work in a diabetes-friendly environment. (see box)

Does your supervisory staff permit you to test your blood sugar and have snacks during the day? Are they threatening to fire you because you have diabetes? If you feel your rights are not being respected, contact the advocacy department of the American Diabetes Association for helpful advice. Their website is *www.diabetes.org* or you can call 1-800-DIABETES.

Eliminate some of the activities that you do

If you volunteer for your church or another worthwhile organization, in addition to all that you do, step back for a while and invite others to do these tasks. If you wish to remain active, take positions that allow you to contribute something unique and important but perhaps take up less of your time. If you run yourself down and cannot care for your health, all who depend on you lose out.

Try yoga or gentle stretching

The style of movement that is taught in several types of yoga can help you recharge your battery, reduce your stress level, and help you deal with the challenges of life with diabetes. There are numerous types of yoga. Some, such as Iyengar and Hatha, are gentle and relaxing. Others, such as Ashtanga, are more athletic and aggressive. Before you sign up for a class, make sure that the style of yoga that is being taught is appropriate for your needs. Let the instructor know if you have any physical issues that may prevent you from participating fully. If you have neuropathy in your feet or hands or any other physical concerns, some of the poses used may not be appropriate for you. There are many websites that can introduce you to the practice of yoga. Two that are very helpful are *www.yogafinder.com* and *www.yogajournal.com*.

Participate in regular physical activity

Exercise releases endorphins and can help relax your muscles and make you feel less stressed. If you are especially stressed in a specific environment, such as your home office, leave the house to do your activity at a health club, community center, or at a park. Invite your loved one to join you and use this time to strengthen your body as well as your relationship. There are various things for a person with diabetes to keep in mind when building an exercise program. A list of risks and recommendations is contained in Table 1, opposite.

Meditate

Meditation is another wonderful stress-reduction tool. It is normally taught by an instructor, but you can try to do it on your own. It can help reduce your stress level, think more clearly, and even lower your blood pressure. All of us would love to come home to a loving partner who is calm and welcoming. Meditate a few minutes before your spouse arrives. As few as 10–20 minutes of quiet breathing can help you shake off a lot of the stress that you have accumulated by the end of the day.

Table 1: Exercising with Diabetic Complications: Risks, Recommendations, and Precautions

	Retinopathy	Nephropathy	Neuropathy	
			Autonomic	Peripheral
Risks	■ Elevations in blood pressure ■ Possible retina detachment from jarring of head	■ Marked changes in hypodynamics ■ Marked elevations in blood pressure ■ Presence of retinopathy likely	■ Hypoglycemia ■ Abnormal blood pressure response ■ Abnormal heart rate response ■ Abnormal thermoregulation (dehydration)	■ Superficial pain ■ Impaired balance/reflexes ■ Numbness/weakness in hands ■ Weakness of thigh muscles
Recommendations	■ Use low-impact activities ■ Monitor blood pressure during exercise ■ Consider stationary cycling, walking, swimming, and low-intensity rowing	■ Include dynamic weight-bearing, low-impact activity ■ Use isometric or light weight lifting when blood pressure is controlled and left ventricular functioning is normal	■ Use submaximal exercise testing ■ Use water activities, stationary cycling, or both	■ Nonweight-bearing activities ■ Use activities that improve balance

Adapted from the *Handbook of Exercise in Diabetes*, American Diabetes Association, 2002.

Positive Effects of Meditation on Stress Relief

Here is a simple type of meditation that you can try right now. It is called focused awareness meditation.

1. Sit in a quiet and comfortable location.
2. Locate an object, such as a candle or a statue that is in your room.
3. With your eyes half-open, gently stare at the object.
4. As you watch the object, focus on your breathing. You can also do this lying down, in a chair, inside, outside, anywhere. It is a very soothing exercise and only requires a few minutes of your time.

Other forms of meditation include mindfulness meditation, which focuses exclusively on breathing, and transcendental meditation, which uses a mantra, or a personal word or phrase that is repeated over and over. You should be able to find a type of meditation that feels right for you.

Listen to relaxing music

Soothing music, especially at bedtime, can help you calm yourself after a challenging day. Invite your partner to listen with you also. Intimacy doesn't happen in the bedroom alone. The time that you spend together, even if it is only in the same room doing different projects, can strengthen your loving bond.

Visit a friend

The support of a friend can also be helpful. Even if you do nothing but laugh or chat about the weather, a meaningful friendship can help change your mood. It can also give you an opportunity to share your daily gripes and groans with someone other than your spouse, especially if you believe that he or she has become tired of listening to them. Don't disclose personal issues without your partner's permission, but you can certainly talk a bit about how challenging life with diabetes can be if your friend welcomes that discussion. This will give you an opportunity to discuss something other than diabetes with your loved one.

Sit outside

We often undervalue the benefit of quiet time. Our world moves so rapidly. Now that we carry cell phones, we are never alone. Take some time to get off of life's treadmill. The fresh air is energizing and the quiet is calming. Some people relax by sitting in front of the television. This can be a helpful break, but many of the disturbing images that come across the screen and upsetting news highlights that are broadcast can change a soothing moment into one of great anxiety.

Enjoy a great book

When is the last time that you sat and enjoyed an engrossing book? The library and bookstore shelves are overflowing with stories that can engage you and take you to a different time and place.

Pamper yourself

Treat yourself to a massage, facial, or manicure. When you feel relaxed and good about your body, you will be more enthusiastic about enjoying intimacy with one you love. The time that you spend engaging in sexual activity should be mutually satisfying for both you and your partner. If you don't feel positively about yourself, it is difficult to relax and fully enjoy the sexual experience.

Schedule intimacy into your life

The connection that you have with your partner can be a great source of support, especially when life becomes hectic. Schedule regular intimate moments with your partner. A weekly evening of bedroom activity or a midday tryst can help boost your spirits and alleviate some of your stress for the remainder of the week. Don't expect your love life to always be spontaneous. Plan ahead and keep it healthy.

Take on new health care behaviors in small, easy-to-do steps

To do this, use the "Jump Start Pledge," which was developed by one of our authors, Janis Roszler. See the Jump Start Pledge box on page 26 for more.

Jump Start Pledge

The Jump Start Pledge is a way to slowly incorporate new health behaviors into your life without becoming overwhelmed. Here is how to do it:

1. Choose a small health behavior.
2. Pledge to do it for a single week.
3. Keep that pledge.
4. At the end of the week, review your progress.
5. Renew the pledge for an additional week, change it, or add another.

Make sure that your pledge is small and easy to accomplish. This will help you build your self-confidence as you improve your overall health and diabetes control.

For example, if you drink five cups of coffee each day and want to cut back on the amount of caffeine that you consume, don't stop suddenly. Your Jump Start Pledge would be to drink four cups rather than five for the next week. You can substitute that cup for a decaffeinated beverage. At the end of your week, if all is well, cut back by an additional cup.

If you had difficulty achieving your initial goal, renew your pledge for another week. As long as you set a Jump Start Pledge each week, you are moving forward toward your ultimate goal of good health.

Seek professional help

If your stress comes from difficulties in your relationship that are more than you can handle on your own, don't hesitate to contact a trained therapist who can help you work them out. To find a qualified therapist in your area, visit *www.aasect.org*, the official site of the American Association of Sex Educators, Counselors, and Therapists.

YOU MAY FEEL ANGRY

In his book, *Diabetes Burnout,* Bill Polonsky, PhD, CDE, coined the term "diabetes police." These are the folks who decide that it is their task to hover over you and correct every diabetes-related move that you make. Although these comments are usually motivated by a combination of love for you and fear for your health, their good intentions rarely come across and can cause you to become quite upset.

Tension From Attempted Weight Loss

"My wife and I used to have a nice relationship. We disagreed now and then, but that happens in all marriages. When I developed type 2 diabetes, Saundra's attitude toward me changed dramatically. She started to nag me constantly about my weight. I tried to lose weight, but really struggled with it. In her opinion, I had caused my diabetes to get even worse. Her friend had type 2 also, but was able to lose weight and control it with diet and exercise. I couldn't do it because I wasn't trying hard enough. I hate her constant nagging. She has turned into some sort of S.W.A.T. team that swoops in whenever I even think about taking a piece of chocolate. Maybe she's correct—I'm not trying hard enough. Maybe I don't care enough about my health and my family. When my diabetes educator asked if we were having any problems in the bedroom, I had to laugh. We are so angry at each other that we now sleep in separate rooms."—*Christopher*

If your spouse has become a diabetes drill sergeant, try the following:

▌ Share how you feel and find out why he or she feels compelled to nag you all of the time. If talking about this issue is difficult, use the "Magic Pencil" exercise described in chapter 7 as a structure for your discussion.

▌ Attend a diabetes class together so you both have up-to-date information about how to care for diabetes. Often, a spouse will nag if he or she believes that you aren't caring for your diabetes properly or aren't taking it seriously enough.

▌ Visit your health care provider together so that you can both hear how he or she wants you to handle certain diabetes-related situations.

YOU MAY WORRY ABOUT BEING REJECTED

Diabetes goes with you wherever you go, including the bedroom. You may feel self-conscious about wearing a pump or worry about the mood swings that you experience when your blood sugar level enters an abnormal range. If you worry about how your mate feels about you and your diabetes, that can carry over into the bedroom where acceptance and communication should be guaranteed. This concern can affect your ability to enjoy and physically react to intimacy.

Keeping Your Diabetes a Secret From Partner

Carl wears an insulin pump. He loves the improved control that he gets with it, but doesn't know what to do in an intimate situation. He read on an Internet message board that some people leave their pump attached to their bodies during sexual activity, but he can't see doing that. Where would it go? He can't picture the logistics of that. He knows that he could disconnect it and leave the small plastic infusion set attached to his abdomen or remove everything and hide the pump somewhere, but can't figure out what to do about the adhesive marks that the infusion set leaves on his skin. He isn't in a committed relationship with anyone who would understand. Sometimes his sexual experiences are with individuals whom he has only known for a short time. Many of them don't even know that he has diabetes. "I don't want to start giving a diabetes lecture when I am alone with someone. That is not how I want to spend my evening!" He is so worried about this.

Dating can be traumatic as well. You may worry that your date will reject you if he or she learns that you have diabetes. Fortunately, some have discovered a way to handle this situation. See Jennifer's story, opposite.

Positive Attitude About Diabetes Boosts Confidence

"I was always afraid to tell my dates about my diabetes. I used to hide it. I didn't want them to think that I was damaged or that any future with me would be filled with doctors and hospitals. Then, it hit me. I was acting damaged, wasn't I? I believed that having diabetes was something to be embarrassed about. It is part of me. Just like my red hair. It is who I am—a great lady who just happens to have diabetes. Now, when I date, I don't flaunt my diabetes, but I don't hide it either. If I have to take a shot, I pull out my pen and inject right through my clothes. No one even notices. If I need to test my blood sugar level, I whip out my meter quickly and do it. I've found that my attitude sets the tone for my date. If I'm relaxed about my diabetes, he will be, too. If I expect any romance to happen, even simple hugging and kissing, I definitely say something. I don't want to suddenly have my blood sugar drop while we are together. And if it does, I want him to understand what the symptoms look like and how he can help me. I just say, if I look a bit drunk or start to act a little strange, my sugar may be going low, so please get me a glass of juice. It doesn't happen often, so don't worry."—*Jennifer*

Poor diabetes control can interfere with many pleasurable activities. If you aren't confident in your diabetes care, speak with your health care team. If they aren't receptive to your needs, seek additional help from a different provider. Don't stop until you are comfortable that you have all of the tools to handle every situation and that you are achieving the best control possible for your diabetes. And also remember to wear medical identification at all times; a card in your wallet isn't enough. It is too easy for you and your wallet or purse to become separated. Low blood sugar symptoms may cause people to believe that you are drunk and need to "sleep it off." If you have a real medical emergency, you want all around you to know that you require medical assistance.

YOU MAY LOSE INTEREST IN SEXUAL ACTIVITIES

Exhaustion Can Ruin a Romantic Evening

Kevin and Tina recently went on a weekend getaway where they expected to relax, use the spa, walk on the beach, and enjoy a generous amount of romance. Their plans changed a bit when the evening rolled around and Kevin chose to hop into bed without Tina. When she peeked into the room, he was sound asleep. "I had hoped that this time away would kindle his interest in sex, but it hasn't made a difference. He has lost interest and I don't know what to do about it." Kevin has had type 2 diabetes for about five years.

Emotional issues

Many emotionally related issues can cause a drop in libido; however, a variety of factors can also affect your sexual interest, including:

■ communication problems within your relationship
■ a lack of romance
■ a hectic schedule that limits time with your partner
■ children and the time required to care for their needs
■ a history of negative or traumatic sexual experiences
■ stress or depression
■ poor self-image from weight gain or other changes

In addition to those listed above, you can also lose interest because of issues that may develop when you have diabetes. How do you feel when your blood sugar is too high or too low? While battling hypoglycemic jitters or high glucose headaches, is it extremely difficult to be in the mood for love.

Financial pressures

Diabetes is expensive, especially if you don't have adequate insurance to cover the test strips, medications, doctor's visits, and other items that you need. Many couples find that diabetes brings significant financial pressures into their lives and into their bedrooms.

Loss of Job Leads to Relationship Problems

"I have type 1 and can't stop the blood sugar roller-coaster ride that I am on. Either I take too little insulin and my blood sugar level soars or I take too much and it plummets. Because of this, I missed a lot of work, so my boss fired me from my position. The loss of my job was rough, but not as rough as the loss of my relationship with my wife. She used to have so much patience with me; I could always count on her. But when my work problems began and money got tight, she started to resent the fact that I had diabetes. Now when I try to hold her, she pulls away. I know that she is angry, but I don't know how to fix things. We now sleep in separate rooms. I feel like I've been fired from my job and my marriage." — *John*

If you feel overwhelmed by the cost of diabetes, speak with your health care team. They should be able to put you in contact with various assistance groups in your local area. A list of pharmaceutical companies with prescription assistance programs are located in the Appendix. Don't let your emotional response to diabetes interfere with your relationships. Take steps to reduce the negative feelings that diabetes has brought into your life.

FOR YOU AND YOUR PARTNER

1 How has diabetes negatively affected how you feel about your sex life, work situation, and day-to-day living?

2 What steps would you like to try to help improve the situation?

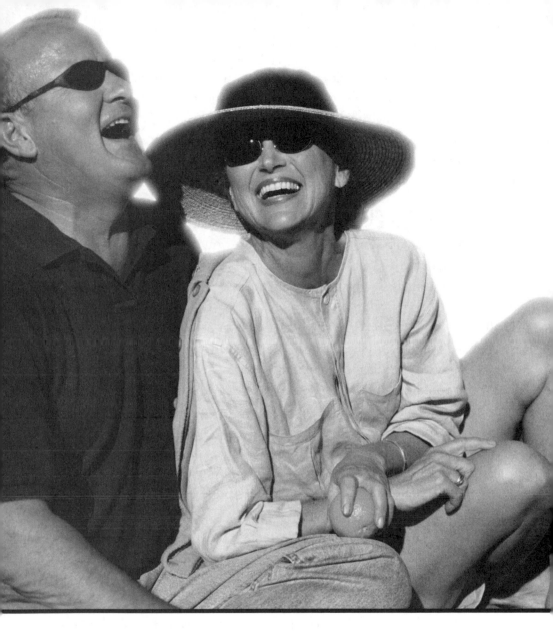

Chapter 3
Diabetes and Your Body

In this chapter:
▪ Explore some of the ways diabetes can affect your body.
▪ Discover several of the things that you can do to help cope with your diabetes.

DIABETES CAN interfere with the intimate physical relationship that you have with your partner. Fortunately, there are many effective treatments available.

Many of the following physical changes that come with diabetes may be familiar to you. After all, you live with your diabetes every day and may have experienced many of them. Let's consider how these symptoms can impact the relationship that you have with your partner.

UNEXPECTED WEIGHT GAIN

Insulin and certain oral medications can cause you to gain weight, which may change how attractive you feel and alter your desire to connect on a physical level with your mate. To help overcome these feelings, try the following:

Follow a healthy weight loss plan

Diabetes meal plans have changed dramatically over the past few years. When you were first diagnosed, you might have been told to avoid all sugar and sugar-containing products. Research has shown that sugar can safely be included in a diabetes meal plan in reasonable amounts. This means that many of the foods that you may have avoided in the past can now be enjoyed in measured portions. Newer, more effective meal planning methods such as carbohydrate counting have also helped individuals fine-tune their weight loss efforts, tame excessive hunger, and improve their diabetes control.

Insulin's Positive and Negative Effects

"After about six years, my type 2 diabetes control became so bad that I had to finally give in and take insulin to help maintain my blood sugar level in a healthier range. The improvement was immediate and impressive. I felt so much better and my blood sugar numbers really started to improve. But then the weight gain began. I now feel so ugly. My clothes keep getting tighter and I hate how I look. To avoid having my husband see how much weight I've gained, I wear looser fitting outfits, change my clothes in private, and head to bed before or after he falls asleep."—*Rhonda*

Here are two popular meal planning options that you might like to try—the Plate Method and carbohydrate counting:

The Plate Method

This meal planning program uses a typical 9-inch dinner plate as a measuring tool. Here is how you use it for your lunch and dinner.

The Plate Method: Lunch/Dinner

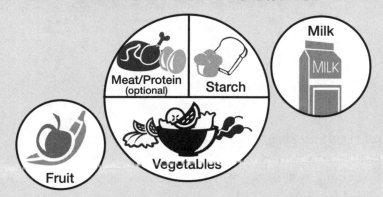

1. Take your plate and mentally draw a line through the center.
2. Fill half of the plate with nonstarchy vegetables. These won't raise your blood sugar level significantly. Nonstarchy vegetables include tomatoes, onions, peppers, celery, lettuce, kale, collard greens, broccoli, cauliflower, zucchini, summer squash, spaghetti squash, green beans, etc. They can also be enjoyed as a soup or vegetable juice.
3. Visually separate the remaining half of your plate into two equal parts. One section is for your protein portion. Protein-rich foods include eggs, meat, cheese, fish, poultry, tofu, and nuts (and should be limited because they contain a significant amount of fat and calories).
4. Place starchy foods in the remaining quarter of the plate, such as rice, bread, pasta, potatoes, sweet potatoes, corn, peas, dry beans, and lentils. Starches and other carb-containing foods provide an important form of energy but can raise your blood sugar level significantly if too many are consumed.
5. Enjoy a small piece of fruit (the size of a tennis ball) or a ½ glass of juice along with the foods that you have placed on your plate.
6. If desired, include an 8-ounce cup of milk (preferably skim) or 1 cup of low-fat yogurt with your meal. If you are not a milk drinker, you can enjoy a serving of starches in place of the milk and take a calcium supplement to help keep your bones healthy.

The Plate Method: Breakfast

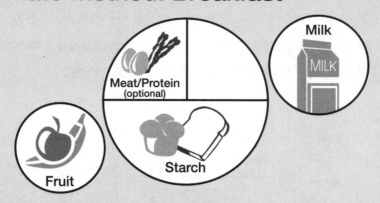

1. Use ¼ to ½ of your plate for your starch serving (bread, cereal, etc.).
2. Enjoy an 8-ounce glass of skim or low-fat milk or 1 cup of low-fat yogurt. If you do not drink milk, replace that serving with an additional portion of starch, as mentioned above.
3. If you wish, you can use ¼ of the plate for an optional protein choice, such as lean sausages, Canadian bacon, or eggs. Include a piece of fruit (tennis ball size), ½ cup of fruit juice, or ¼ cup dried fruit.

The Plate Method offers lots of flexibility. You can eat in any restaurant or at anyone's home; just place the appropriate food choices on your plate in the areas mentioned above. For additional information, visit *www.platemethod.com*.

Carbohydrate counting

This method of meal planning requires you to identify carbohydrate-containing foods and estimate the amount that you plan to eat. The easiest way to know how many carbohydrates are in a particular food is to use the information located on its Nutrition Facts label (see opposite).

Watch your food portions

Restaurants today offer portions that are far larger than ever existed in the past. While out, you can easily estimate food portions with your hands. Several of the measurements are listed on p. 38.

Nutrition Facts

Serving Size 1/2 cup (114g)
Servings Per Container 4

Amount Per Serving

Calories 90   Calories from Fat 30

	% Daily Value*
Total Fat 3g	**5%**
Saturated Fat 0g	**0%**
Cholesterol 0mg	**0%**
Sodium 300mg	**13%**
Total Carbohydrate 13g	**4%**
Dietary Fiber 3g	**12%**
Sugars 3g	
Protein 3g	

Vitamin A 80%   •   Vitamin C 60%

Calcium 10%   Iron 10%

* Percent Daily Values are based on a 2,000 calorie diet. Your daily values may be higher or lower depending on your calorie needs:

	Calories:	2,000	2,500
Total Fat	Less than	65g	80g
Sat Fat	Less than	20g	25g
Cholesterol	Less than	300mg	300mg
Sodium	Less than	2,400mg	2,400mg
Total Carbohydrate		300g	375g
Dietary Fiber		25g	30g

Calories per gram:
Fat 9 • Carbohydrate 4 • Protein 4

1. Find the serving size at the top of the label. All of the information included on the label is for this particular serving amount. If you eat twice as much, double the nutrition information. If you eat half of that amount, cut the nutrition values in half. The label to the left states that the serving size of this item is ½ cup.

2. Search for the **Total Carbohydrate** amount that is given. It is highlighted in bold lettering. That is the amount of carbohydrates found in one serving of this food. Our sample label shows that this item contains 13 grams of carbohydrates. Beneath the **Total Carbohydrate**, you will find additional details about this category that are not printed in bold. Ignore the sugar amount, as it is already included in the carbohydrate total. If you are just beginning to count your carbohydrates, you can start here. Once you feel more comfortable with this method, add the following two steps.

3. Check the dietary fiber amount that is listed. If it is greater than 5 grams, deduct it from the total carbohydrate amount. Fiber does not affect your blood sugar level. In our sample label, the product contains 3 grams of dietary fiber, so you don't have to deduct this amount.

4. Consider the sugar alcohol content. If an item contains any of this sweetener, it will be listed beneath the **Total Carbohydrate** amount. Take half of that amount and add it to the **Total Carbohydrate**. Sugar alcohols raise blood sugar levels, but not as much as sugar will. That is why you only add half.

To learn more about carbohydrate counting, read *Guide to Carb Counting, 2nd edition*, by Hope Warshaw and Karmeen Kulkarni (ADA, 2004). A great source for carbohydrate information is *www.calorieking.com*. It contains the nutrient content of many different foods.

Easy Portion Estimations

Palm of your hand = 3 ounces. Use this measurement to estimate cooked meat or fish. A 3-ounce piece should be approximately the size and thickness of your palm minus your fingers and thumb.

A tightly held fist = ½ cup. This can help you estimate a serving of pasta or rice. It is also a reasonable serving of cut fruit.

A cupped hand = 1 cup. If you wish to estimate a single cup of vegetables or noodles, estimate with this measurement.

The tip of your thumb = 1 teaspoon. Use this measurement to estimate fatty condiments, such as mayonnaise or margarine.

Your entire thumb = 1 Tablespoon. The distance that runs from the tip of your thumb down to your second knuckle can help you estimate salad dressing or any item that you'd like to keep limited to a single tablespoon.

Your first two fingers = 1 ounce. A single ounce of cheese or meat can be measured easily by matching it to the length and width of your two fingers when they are held together.

Consume a healthy amount of fiber

Fiber-rich foods can help fill you up so that you are better able to meet your weight goals and may help control your blood sugar levels by slowing down digestion. Increase your fiber intake slowly or you may experience some unpleasant gastrointestinal discomfort and flatulence. Here are the 10 best sources of fiber in different food categories.

Best Sources of Fiber

STARCHES	Serving	Fiber (g)
Bran cereal (for example: All Bran, 100% Bran, Bran Buds, Fiber One)	½ cup	10–18
Acorn Squash, boiled or baked	1 cup	7–11

STARCHES (continued)	Serving	Fiber (g)
Butternut squash	1 cup	6–7
Dried beans, peas, lentils	½ cup	5–8
Bran Flake cereals	¾ cup	4–6
Rye wafer cracker	4	5
Peas, green, frozen, boiled	½ cup	5
Bulgur, cooked	½ cup	4
Corn, cooked	½ cup, 1 (5-oz) cob	4
Air popped popcorn	3 cups	4
VEGETABLES	**Serving**	**Fiber (g)**
Brussels sprouts, cooked	½ cup	4
Artichoke	½	3
Spinach, cooked	½ cup	3
Broccoli, cooked	½ cup	3
Jicama, raw	½ cup	3
Pea pods/snow peas, cooked	½ cup	2
Okra, cooked	½ cup	2
Green beans, cooked	½ cup	2
Tomato products	1 serving	2
FRUITS	**Serving**	**Fiber (g)**
Red raspberries	1 cup	5
Blackberries	¾ cup	5
Blueberries	¾ cup	4
Strawberries	1 ¼ cups	3
Prunes	3	3
Dried apricots	8 halves	3
Dried figs	1 ½	3
Apple	1 small	3
Orange	1 small	2
Pear	½ large fresh	2

The Diabetes Food & Nutrition Bible, by Hope Warshaw, MMSc, RD, CDE, and Robyn Webb, MS

To help you update your current eating plan, meet with a registered dietitian in your area. To find one, contact your local hospital or visit *www.eatright.org*, the official website of the American Dietetic Association.

Try what has worked for others

The National Weight Control Registry (NWCR) was established in 1994 by Rena Wing, PhD, from Brown Medical School, and James O. Hill, PhD, from the University of Colorado, and is the largest study of long-term successful weight loss maintenance. It records the behaviors of individuals who have successfully maintained a weight loss of over 30 pounds for at least one year. The following are some of the eating behaviors that worked for many of the folks they interviewed.

1994 NWCR Weight Loss Maintenance Study Results

- 93.6% restrict their intake of certain high-sugar and high-fat foods.
- 78% eat breakfast each day.
- 50% rely heavily on portion control.
- 39% limit their fat intake.
- 36% count their calories.

The participants use numerous weight loss techniques. Many lost weight on their own, but the majority participated in commercial programs and self-help groups and used the help of registered dietitians and psychologists. To maintain their loss, they weighed themselves regularly, limited their restaurant visits to less than three times per week, and participated in regular physical activity. To be part of this registry or to get additional information, visit *www.nwcr.ws* or call 1-800-606-NWCR.

Review your diabetes medications with your health care team

There are many different diabetes medications to choose from. If one is causing you to gain extra weight, try another. You might be able to use Byetta or Symlin, two new medications to help you tackle this problem.

Byetta

Byetta has a fascinating story. When young endocrinologist Dr. John Eng learned that several new digestive hormones had been identified by researchers at the National Institutes of Health and medical institutes in Belgium and Sweden, he was determined to uncover the role they played in digestion. His research led him to a strange discovery—the Gila monster's saliva contained a substance that could help people with type 2 diabetes improve their blood sugar control. A Gila monster eats four times a year. Between feedings, his body stops releasing insulin. When it is time for another feeding, his body produces exenatide, which restarts its insulin production.

Exenatide is very similar to the human hormone GLP-l. Individuals who have type 2 diabetes do not produce adequate amounts of this hormone. Byetta contains a synthetic version of exenatide, which

∎ helps the pancreas release additional insulin.
∎ slows down the rate at which the body absorbs food.
∎ helps you feel full more quickly.
∎ decreases the amount of glucose that the liver produces.
∎ encourages weight loss in many people who take it.

Byetta can be used by people who take metformin, a sulfonylurea, or a combination of the two of them.

Symlin

Symlin is an analogue of a similar hormone found in the body and is released by the same cell that produces insulin. It plays a dual role—helping to control the way your body handles blood sugars and signals the brain's satiety center—so you will recognize that you are being fed. This message is important for successful weight control. People with type 1 or type 2 who take mealtime insulin can use Symlin. Many have successfully lost weight and kept it off by adding this new medication to their diabetes care plan.

Treat your blood sugar lows appropriately

Many people overtreat their hypoglycemia episodes and gain unwanted weight. If you experience a low blood sugar episode, don't grab a container and drink generous amounts of orange juice or eat fistfuls of candy until your hypoglycemic symptoms disappear. Examples of hypoglycemia symptoms are:

▌ headache
▌ shakiness
▌ sweating
▌ fatigue
▌ irritability

Your glucose level will normalize before the symptoms finally go away. If you eat or drink until those unpleasant feelings disappear, you will consume unneeded calories, send your blood sugar level back up, and gain weight. Instead, use the 15/15 Rule when your blood sugar level is below 70 mg/dl or below your target range.

The 15/15 Rule

1. Eat 15 grams of a fast-acting carbohydrate.*
2. Wait 15 minutes.
3. Test again.
4. If your level remains low, repeat steps 1, 2, and 3. If your level is above 70 mg/dl or within your target range, stop eating.

*Servings that contain 15 grams of fast-acting carbohydrate include:

▌ ½ cup of fruit juice
▌ 3–4 glucose tablets (read package)
▌ ½ can of regular soda (not diet)
▌ 2 Tablespoons of raisins
▌ 5 LifeSavers candies
▌ 1 Tablespoon granulated sugar or honey

Eat a healthy amount of carbohydrates

Excessively low-carbohydrate diets are popular, but can be unhealthy. Your body uses carbohydrate-containing foods for energy. When these aren't available, it turns to fat and protein, which don't burn efficiently. When fat is metabolized, it releases undesirable by-products called ketones. They can make you feel lightheaded and even nauscous. Extremely high levels of ketones in the body can be life threatening. The American Diabetes Association suggests that you consume at least 130 grams of carbohydrates each day. This is the amount needed to meet the needs of your brain and central nervous system. Less than that is not recommended.

Drink plenty of water

There is a debate about how much water a person should consume each day, but one fact is not in dispute—water fills you up and can help you eat less. Drink a large glass of water before you sit down to a meal. It will make you feel full and help you overcome the urge to overeat. If you feel hungry between meals, drink some water first and then see if you are still hungry. We eat for a variety of reasons in addition to actual hunger. We may snack while nervous, bored, or just out of habit. If you aren't truly hungry, a glass of water can help appease that need to eat foods that you really don't desire.

Stay physically active

Exercise can have many positive effects on your lifestyle and your health. It can

- help you reach your weight goals.
- improve your insulin sensitivity.
- improve your A1C level.
- encourage better cholesterol.
- help you feel fit.
- develop the body shape that you desire.

Find an activity that you enjoy, such as dancing, fencing, biking, or swimming. If you don't like to exercise, invite your spouse to join you and turn your workout into a date. Sexual activity is also a physical activity and can count as part of your daily workout as well.

When you exercise, do it safely. Start slowly and gently build up to a greater intensity of 30–45 minutes, 3–5 days per week, when possible. To encourage weight loss, you may have to increase your activity level to at least one hour of moderate activity, such as walking, or 30 minutes of vigorous activity, such as jogging.

To make sure that you aren't overdoing your exercise, take the talk test. If you are able to carry on a conversation without becoming too winded, you are doing fine. In chapter 7, we will discuss different ways for you to enhance your relationship with your partner. Inviting him or her to join you as you workout, is certainly a great way to accomplish that goal.

De-emphasize your weight

Your loved one hopefully chose you for more than your outward appearance. Remember that your connection is more than just a physical one. Discuss your weight concerns with your partner and see if it does bother him or her. You may assume that your spouse feels a particular way that may not be correct. If your weight makes certain sexual positions less comfortable, be creative and try different ones. There are numerous books that can provide you with a wealth of different sexual options including the old favorite, *The Joy of Sex*, by Alex Comfort. If your weight becomes an issue that you can't overcome, it may be helpful to discuss your concerns with a qualified counselor. Ask your health care team for a recommendation.

You may develop nerve damage

When you were a child, did you ever create a telephone by tying two paper cups to a string? You held a cup at your end and your friend held his cup at the other. As the string was pulled taut, you'd whisper your secret message into the cup and your words would magically travel to the other end. If the line was relaxed or cut, you could continue talking, but your message would not reach its destination. Like the string on your childhood phone, your nerves communicate messages back and forth from your brain to the other areas of your body. If any nerves are damaged by exposure to high blood sugar levels for a sustained period of time (months or years), the signal sent by your brain will be weakened or interrupted. This means that the message that is sent to start an erection or have a woman's body lubricate may not reach its destination.

Blood glucose goals

The following are suggested blood glucose goals for men and women with diabetes from the American Diabetes Association. Yours may differ. Review your personal blood glucose needs with your health care providers.

Blood glucose goals

A1C:	Below 7% for most individuals, or as close to normal (less than 6%) as possible for those who can achieve it without significant hypoglycemia
Before meals:	between 90 and 130 mg/dl
1–2 hours after the first bite of a meal:	below 180 mg/dl

American Diabetes Association Clinical Practice Recommendations, 2007

To help improve your control, check your blood sugar level at specific times throughout the day. Your physician may have asked you to test before your meals and at bedtime. This information helps your health care team assess your diabetes care plan. If you test 1–2 hours after you take the first bite of a meal, you can observe how your food choices affect your diabetes control. If your blood sugar level after lunch is greater than 180 mg/dl, you may need to reduce your carbohydrate portion, increase your medication, or increase your physical activity level.

ED and Diabetes: Wake-Up Call

Douglas knew that he had type 2 diabetes, but ignored it. He liked what he ate and ate what he liked. He didn't make any effort to exercise and never checked his blood sugar level; he didn't even own a glucose monitor. When the nurse at his doctor's office offered him a free one to use at home, he refused. What finally changed his attitude was an article about erectile dysfunction that caught his eye while waiting to see his doctor. Douglas was surprised to learn that diabetes could affect him in the bedroom. That changed everything. He quickly called the doctor's office and made an appointment to learn how to use a monitor.

When you check your blood, you receive important information, but it is far from complete. Your results only provide you with a snapshot of your blood sugar level at that single moment in time. You don't know if your level is going up or going down. You don't know what your level is while asleep or at other times of the day. Fortunately, your A1C value offers this missing information. It represents your average blood glucose level for the past 2–3 months. If it is below 7% and you feel good, your risk of developing diabetes-related sexual complications (and other complications) should be low. To better understand your A1C value, locate it on the chart below and check out its mg/dl equivalent, the type of result that appears on your glucose meter.

Determining Average Blood Glucose for the Past Few Months

A1C level (%)	Glucose equivalent (mg/dl)
6	135
7	170
8	205
9	240
10	275
11	310
12	345

Here is an example of how to use this chart: If your A1C level is 9%, your average blood glucose level for the past 2–3 months was approximately 240 mg/dl. If it was 11%, your glucose level has been approximately 310 mg/dl for the last few months. An A1C of less than 7% puts you at a lower risk for complications.

American Diabetes Association Clinical Practice Recommendations, 2007

YOU MAY HAVE CIRCULATION PROBLEMS

Blood flow plays an essential role in sexual response. To become fully erect, a penis fills with about 11 times the amount of blood that it normally contains. A woman's clitoris will enlarge when additional blood becomes trapped inside. Her skin may also redden over much of her body as an increased amount of blood flows to the skin. If any vessels are blocked or narrowed, which happens more frequently when diabetes is present, it will take longer for the blood to reach its destination.

Good circulation requires a healthy heart and blood vessels. To achieve this, participate in some form of physical activity on a regular basis—including sexual activity—maintain a healthy blood pressure, and keep your blood vessels open and clear.

Most experts recommend that people with diabetes maintain a blood pressure of less than 130/80. If your blood pressure is too high or too low, your blood flow will be affected.

Recommended Blood Pressure for Diabetics—130/80

The top number, 130, represents the systolic pressure. That is the amount of force that is used to squeeze the heart and send blood throughout the body.

The bottom number, 80, is the diastolic pressure. This is the amount of force that the heart uses when it relaxes between each contraction.

Abnormal blood pressure

Unlike blood sugar highs and lows, abnormal blood pressure is not always accompanied by symptoms. If your doctor has prescribed blood pressure medication, take it even if you feel well. There are many medications that can help you return your blood pressure to a normal level. They include calcium channel blockers, diuretics, angiotensin-converting enzymes (ACE inhibitors), angiotensin receptor blockers (ARBs), and Beta blockers.

Blood Pressure Medications

▮ Beta blockers—help the heart beat with less force.
▮ Calcium channel blockers—help the blood vessels relax by preventing the entry of calcium into the heart and bloodstream.
▮ Diuretics (water pills)—enable the body to rid itself of excess sodium and fluid. When these levels are high, they force the heart to work harder.
▮ ACE inhibitors (angiotensin-converting enzyme) and ARBs (angiotensin receptor blockers) prevent the hormone angiotensin from narrowing your blood vessels.

Excessive lipids in your bloodstream can also impede the flow of blood to the sexual organs. The types of lipids (fats) that are particularly problematic are cholesterol, triglycerides, saturated fats, and trans fats.

Cholesterol

Cholesterol is found in animal products, such as:
▮ high-fat cheeses
▮ fatty meats
▮ 2% and whole milk
▮ egg yolks
▮ butter
▮ ice cream

Your body produces cholesterol as well and comes in two forms: HDL and LDL. The LDL, or "bad," cholesterol is sticky and adheres to the inside of blood vessels. When this occurs, the vessel passageways become narrowed. HDL, or "good," cholesterol helps remove LDL cholesterol from the body. As you can guess, a high level of HDL is preferable. The amount of triglycerides (fat) that you have in your blood will climb if you consume too many oils, carbohydrates, or alcohol.

Target Goals for Cholesterol

The American Diabetes Association recommends the following target goals for cholesterol and triglycerides:

HDL	Greater than 40 mg/dl (1.1 mmol/l)
LDL	Less than 100 mg/dl (2.6 mmol/l)
Triglycerides	Less than 150 mg/dl (1.7 mmol/l)

American Diabetes Association: Clinical Practice Recommendations, 2007

Saturated fats and trans fats can affect circulation and increase the risk of heart disease. They raise bad LDL cholesterol levels and are primarily found in the fat that comes from animal products, such as poultry, whole milk, and meats. Nonanimal sources include coconut and palm oils and palm kernel oil. Your intake of saturated fats should be limited. Trans fats are created when manufacturers take liquid vegetable oils and add hydrogen to make them more solid, which improves their use in baking. They should be limited as well, because they not only raise the bad LDL cholesterol level, they lower your good HDL cholesterol level. The Nutrition Facts labels found on different food products now indicate if an item contains trans fats.

If your lipid level is high, reduce it by trying the following:

- Eat less fat of all types.
- Reduce your alcohol intake.
- Eat fewer sweets.
- Lose weight.
- Improve your blood glucose control.
- Increase your physical activity level.
- Stop smoking.
- Reduce your carbohydrate intake, especially refined carbs such as white rice, white pasta, and white bread.
- Eat more fiber—whole grains, fruits, and vegetables.

YOU MAY DEVELOP BRUISES

Preventing Bruising During Injections

To help keep bruises from appearing after you inject insulin or another diabetes-related medication, try the following:

1. Pinch your skin before injecting.
2. Touch the needle very lightly to the skin and slowly push it in.
3. Pull back immediately if you feel any pain. You may be touching a blood vessel, which will cause bruising if pierced.

Move the needle over slightly and try again. You can also switch to an insulin pen, which uses a smaller needle.

YOU MIGHT HAVE PERSONAL HYGIENE ISSUES

Poorly controlled diabetes can cause bad breath, dry and itchy skin, and sweating. When you don't eat an adequate amount of carbohydrates or your body is unable to use them as its primary source of energy, it will break down fat and protein. As it metabolizes fat, ketones are released, causing an unpleasant, fruity breath odor.

When blood glucose levels climb too high, the body rids itself of the excess amount by producing additional urine. This can cause your skin to become dehydrated, dry, and itchy. Diabetes-related nerve damage can also cause the body to sweat excessively, especially around the face and torso. To help prevent these problems from developing, eat a reasonable amount of carbohydrates each day and take enough medication, if needed, to utilize them properly for energy. Drink plenty of fluids and keep your blood sugar level within a normal range.

Diabetes can cause changes to occur that may affect your ability to enjoy intimacy. Let's continue to review additional treatments that you can use to try to improve this situation.

FOR YOU AND YOUR PARTNER

1 Identify ways that diabetes has affected your body.

2 Have you shared these changes with your health care professional? If not, why not?

3 How can you support each other when these problems arise?

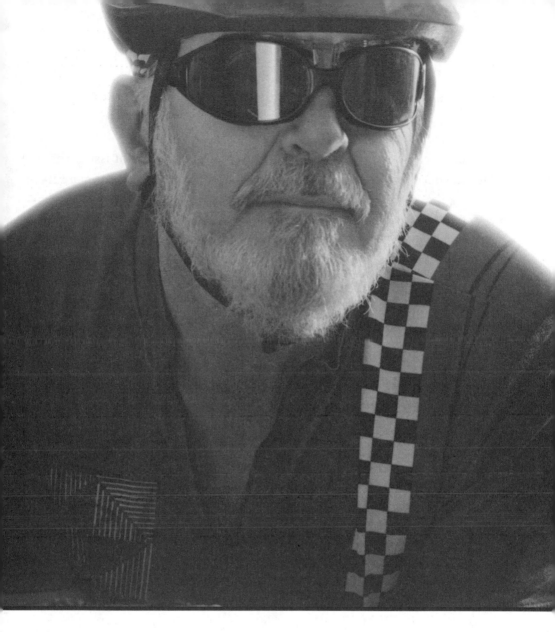

Chapter 4
For Him

In this chapter:
▮ Learn more about erectile dysfunction.
▮ Explore a variety of treatment options.

IF YOU ARE A MAN with diabetes, at some point in your life you may have difficulty achieving and maintaining a successful erection or your desire for sex may change. Fortunately, there are many effective treatments that can help.

In the previous chapters, we provided a general overview of issues that could make it more challenging for both men and women to enjoy a fulfilling sex life. This chapter is focused on you specifically—a man with diabetes. The most common sexual side effect in men is erectile dysfunction, also referred to as "ED."

ERECTILE DYSFUNCTION

At some time in their lives, most men will have some difficulty developing or sustaining an erection. Although it is upsetting, it is quite common and is not usually cause for concern. The problem is considered ED when a man is unable to achieve and maintain an erection sufficient enough to enjoy the sexual experience in more than half of his attempts. This problem used to be called "impotence," but that term is outdated and unfair. Impotence implies that a man is no longer a successful male in all areas of his life. Men with ED can still be successful businessmen, athletes, fathers, partners, and friends.

Diabetes is not the only cause of ED. It can also develop from the following:

▌ Illegal drugs, such as marijuana and cocaine, which alter the body's ability to function properly.

▌ Emotional difficulties, such as anxiety, stress, and depression. If you feel negatively about something, that emotion can translate into problems in the bedroom.

▌ Medication—this topic will be discussed in greater detail later in this chapter.

▌ Prostate surgery—any surgical procedure in the genital area can affect your body's ability to perform sexually. In many cases, this is a temporary change. Discuss this concern with your health care team.

▌ Radiation therapy—any type of treatment that focuses on the genital area can have an effect.

▌ Injury

▌ The diabetes-related physical concerns that were presented in chapter 3.

Erectile Dysfunction

Prevalence of ED in General Population: 4–9% (estimated)

Prevalence of ED in Men with Diabetes:

	AGE	PREVALENCE
	20–29	9%
	Over 30	15%
Under 30 with 10 years of diabetes		20%
	60 or older	55%
	Over 70	95%

AADE—New Perspectives on Erectile Dysfunction

DIABETES AND YOUR MEDICATION

As a man with diabetes, you may need to take certain medications to treat or prevent diabetic complications. Some of them may encourage the development of erection problems. A partial list of these medicines that was compiled by *Healthwise* (2004) is located in the Appendix. If you have ED, evaluate your medicine choices with your health care team.

DIABETES AND YOUR HORMONE LEVELS

If you have already tried Viagra or one of the other pills without success or can't pinpoint the exact cause of your erection problems, your ED may be caused by a low testosterone ("Low T") level. Men with diabetes are more than twice as likely to have Low T compared to other men. Those who have low levels may experience:

▌ decreased sex drive
▌ erectile dysfunction
▌ depression
▌ fatigue

An estimated 13 million American men age 45 and older have this problem, yet fewer than 10% seek treatment. Fortunately, Low T can be easily treated.

Testosterone is a hormone that promotes hair growth, muscle development, bone health, sperm production, and helps you maintain a healthy sexual appetite. If you are overweight or have high blood pressure, your risk for developing Low T will increase.

Symptoms of Low T include:

- decreased sex drive
- erectile dysfunction
- depression
- fatigue
- weight gain (increased fat)
- drop in bone mineral density
- reduced strength and muscle mass

These symptoms are easily confused with other medical symptoms, which is one reason why Low T is often undiagnosed. A simple blood test that is taken in the morning can confirm if this is an issue for you. Testosterone levels normally peak in the morning, so the test is usually run at that time. If your level is below normal, there are several very effective treatments that can help.

Gels

In a study published in the *Journal of Urology*, a group of 75 men with low levels of testosterone experienced a 34% improvement in their sexual performance when they used a testosterone gel along with Viagra. It is an easy option to use and has very encouraging results.

Patches

Hormone patches can be placed onto the shoulders, abdomen, or upper arms and are worn for a period of 24 hours. The patches may cause itching or blisters. If this happens to you, report the reaction to your physician.

Injections

It is also possible to increase your testosterone level with an injection that is provided by your doctor every 7–21 days.

Oral (buccal) tablets

Another option is a testosterone-containing tablet that is placed onto the inside of the cheek. It is left there for a period of 12 hours.

Let's review the pros and cons of several ED options and hear what several patients learned by using them.

Testosterone Gel Is an Easy Fix for Low T

Ben is 35 and has had type 1 diabetes for 24 years. Several years ago, he developed depression and erectile dysfunction. When sex did occur, it was not satisfying for him or for his wife. His wife tried to be more appealing by wearing new lingerie, but that just put additional pressure on him to perform, which he was unable to do. He always prided himself on being a man who could satisfy his wife. Suddenly he was unable to do that and became very frustrated. He and his wife started to fight and their marriage became stressed. Fortunately for Ben, he had a doctor who decided to test his testosterone level, which was low. He started treatment with a testosterone gel that he applied to his shoulders once a day. Within two to four weeks, life took a significant turn for the better. "I felt like a new man. I was happy and motivated again and within another couple of months had my sex drive back. I never would have believed that a hormone issue could have such an effect on my family life. I also had no idea that a simple gel could help me regain my ability to be sexually active again."

Could It Be Low T?

To see if you are at risk for low testosterone, answer "yes" or "no" to the following questions. Choose the response that best describes how you have been feeling.

1. Do you have a decrease in libido (sex drive)? ☐ Yes ☐ No
2. Do you have a lack of energy? ☐ Yes ☐ No
3. Do you have a decrease in strength and/or endurance? ☐ Yes ☐ No
4. Have you lost height? ☐ Yes ☐ No
5. Have you noticed a decreased "enjoyment of life"? ☐ Yes ☐ No
6. Are you sad and/or grumpy? ☐ Yes ☐ No
7. Are your erections less strong? ☐ Yes ☐ No
8. Have you noticed deterioration in your ability to play sports? ☐ Yes ☐ No
9. Are you falling asleep after dinner? ☐ Yes ☐ No
10. Has there been deterioration in your work performance? ☐ Yes ☐ No

If you answer "yes" to questions 1 or 7, or "yes" to three or more of the other questions, then you may be a candidate for a blood test. Be sure to discuss the results of this quiz with your diabetes educator and doctor.

Source: *www.diabeteseducator.org* (Morley JE, Charlton E, Patrick P, et al. Validation of a screening questionnaire for androgen deficiency in aging males. *Metabolism.* 2000; 40:1239–1242)

ORAL MEDICATIONS

There are currently three oral medications available to treat ED—Viagra (sildenafil), Levitra (vardenafil HCL), and Cialis (tadalafil). Viagra was the first oral medication for ED approved by the FDA. It is the "little blue pill" that, with the help of Senator Bob Dole, heightened the public awareness of ED.

If you enjoy having alcohol as a prelude to intimate activity, you are permitted to do so as long as you drink in moderation.

There are a few conditions that you should be aware of if you choose to use any of these pills. They should not be used with any medications that contain nitrates or with an alpha blocker, such as Hytrin or Cardura. (Cialis can be used with the alpha blocker Flomax). The nitrate that is

ED Medications and Their Effectiveness

Pills are effective in 50–60% of all men with diabetes. They can be used every day, if desired, and are very simple to use.

▮ Viagra begins working within 15–30 minutes and stays active for up to four hours.

▮ Levitra begins working within 10–30 minutes and stays active for up to 12 hours.

▮ Cialis begins working within 15 minutes and stays active for up to 36 hours.

found in foods is not a concern when taking these medications. You should avoid taking them after eating a high-fat meal or their absorption will be delayed. They may also cause your erection to last longer than four hours. If that occurs, you should contact your physician.

Side effects of oral medications may include:

▮ mild flushing ▮ headache ▮ upset stomach
▮ back pain ▮ muscle aches ▮ stuffy nose
▮ dizziness

They may also cause you to see a blue-green tinge or become sensitive to light. This is temporary and goes away when the medication wears off. Also take care to stand up slowly after intimate activity. This will help you reduce or avoid the chance that you may become dizzy.

Making the Most of Preparation Time

"When I received my prescription for Levitra, I was told that I should take it about an hour before my wife and I have sex and while we wait, I should do something that is sexually stimulating like read an adult magazine, watch a suggestive video, or enjoy foreplay with my partner. My wife and I get pretty creative with this waiting period and have lots of fun."—*David*

Injections

The medication that is used for injection is known as Caverject (alprostadil), which, like oral medication, relaxes muscle tissue and dilates the blood vessels in the penis to encourage the movement of blood into the penis. It is easily mixed by the user, injected directly into the penis, and stimulates an erection very quickly. Caverject has an interesting origin. A form of this drug was originally used to help dilate the heart valves in small babies so that their blood would flow easier. Researchers who focused their efforts on erection problems found that this drug could also help blood flow in men to help create an erection.

If you haven't had success with any other product, penile injections may work for you. They are effective in 70–90% of men, create a strong erection within approximately 10–15 minutes, and can last up to one hour. The downside of this option is that it can only be used every other day for a maximum of three times per week and may eventually cause scarring

Penile Injections

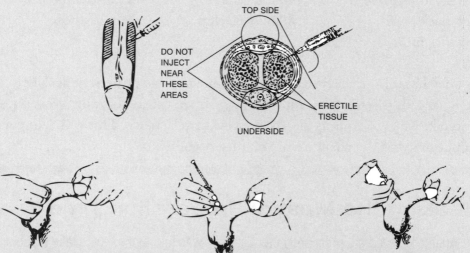

Vince didn't want to wait up to an hour to achieve a response, so he opted to skip the pills and try something else. The idea of injecting his penis initially caused him to hesitate, but the reward of having a quick and effective erection made it worthwhile.

or pain. As with the pills that were listed above, it is possible to develop a sustained erection that will require medical attention.

Penile Injection Tips

"Although it is very tempting, I learned that I shouldn't inject more than the recommended dose of medication; my friend tried it and needed medical help to get his erection to end. I learned to inject myself at a 60-degree angle from the top center area of the penis. It was surprisingly easy to do, especially while sitting down. Like insulin, I also learned that it is important to rotate injection sites to prevent scarring."—*Vince*

Suppositories

A year before Viagra hit the market, Muse, the first penile alprostadil suppository treatment for ED, appeared on the scene. It gave hope and promise to many men as the first noninjectable option available for ED. The suppository is about the size of a grain of rice and is housed in a small applicator that is inserted into the tip of the penis. As with injected alprostadil, this medication relaxes the muscles and dilates blood vessels so blood can flow more easily into the penis.

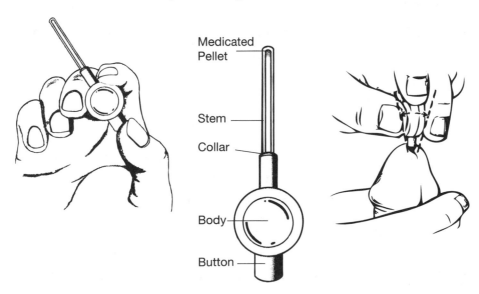

Medicated Pellet

Stem

Collar

Body

Button

Penile suppositories should be inserted 10–15 minutes prior to intimate activity. An erection should develop within 10–20 minutes. They can be used twice daily and are successful in about 35% of the men who try them. Unlike the oral agents, suppositories can be used if you take nitroglycerin. The downside to this form of treatment is that they are very expensive and can cause testicular pain, dizziness, burning and irritation after insertion, and pain in the scrotal area or upper thighs. You should avoid participating in oral sexual activity while using this treatment and may need to wear a condom if your partner experiences burning from this medication or is pregnant.

Easy to Use

"I found the suppository very easy to use. My educator showed me how to do it and it works. Just be sure to urinate before you insert it—it helps lubricate the passageway inside of the penis. It also helps to walk around and massage the area until the pellet dissolves. I was told that the suppository could cause my partner to feel an unpleasant burning sensation, so I wore a condom, which worked really well."—*Jerry*

Devices

There are also several ED treatment tools available that require no prescription and are easy to obtain. They include:

■ constriction bands
■ vacuum pumps
■ penile support sleeves

Many can be purchased over the counter and some insurance plans will cover their cost if you obtain them with a physician's prescription. You probably won't see these items sitting on the shelf at a local pharmacy, but can order them from most pharmacy Internet sites. They are also available from medical supply stores. Be wary of the versions that are sold at local sex shops. Some may be adequate, but others may not be made well and are a waste of time and money.

A Variety of Treatment Options

David arrived at his doctor's office to ask for a prescription for Viagra. He had seen it on several commercials and assumed that it was the best drug to try. Fortunately, his physician presented him with a variety of different choices, including several devices that he could purchase with or without a prescription. He was pleased to learn that he had options; that he could choose a treatment that would fit into his lifestyle.

"I was happy to learn that I could use a different treatment if one didn't suit me or work to my satisfaction. Choice is a good thing."

Constriction rings

The constriction ring holds the blood in place once it has entered the penis. If you are able to develop an erection, but have difficulty maintaining it, this option may be a good one for you. Think of a balloon—it will stay inflated as long as the end is held tightly enough to prevent air from escaping. Once the penis becomes erect, stretch the constriction ring over the top of the penis and slide it down to the base. Like a rubber band, the ring holds blood inside the penis until it is removed.

Constriction rings are very simple to use. They are inexpensive and don't have to affect the spontaneity of any intimate moment, especially if you have an enthusiastic partner who is willing to incorporate it into your foreplay. When you use the ring, several things will happen that you should be aware of—the penis will stay erect, but it may be a bit wobbly at the base and it may develop a bluish color change. Have you ever wrapped a rubber band around your finger? It cuts off the blood flow and your skin begins to turn a darker color. That is what you are doing with the constriction ring—you are putting a significant amount of pressure on one area so that blood flow stops. Because the warm flow of blood is not entering into the penis, your skin may feel cool to the touch. That is normal, so don't worry. Once you've removed the ring, your color and warm temperature will return.

It isn't wise to leave the constriction ring in place for longer than 30 minutes. Don't fall asleep while wearing it. Your skin may be a bit tender

More Options to Fit Every Need

"When it comes to constriction rings, size does matter. Try different sized rings until you find the one that works for you." —*Xavier*

when you remove the ring and it is possible that the ring will pull off a few strands of hair as it comes off. To help prevent this, rub the area with pre-warmed lubricant before you remove it.

If you have difficulty sliding on a constriction ring, you can use a tool known as a "penile tourniquet." A ring can also be used with a vacuum pump (which will be discussed in a moment). That combination will enhance your erection.

Vacuum pump

The vacuum pump is a great choice for most men. It is made up of a plastic cylinder, a handheld or battery-operated pump, water-soluble lubricant, and a set of constriction rings.

Instructions for Using a Vacuum Pump

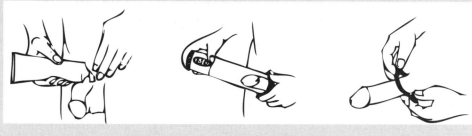

1. Place the constriction ring onto the cylinder as directed.
2. Lubricate your flaccid (not erect) penis with a generous amount of lubricant.
3. Put the cylinder over the penis and hold the cylinder tightly against your abdomen. As you activate the pump it creates a vacuum within the tube that draws blood into the penis.

Once it is erect, the constriction ring is slipped off the cylinder and secured around the base of the penis to prevent the blood from leaving.

There are several benefits to using a vacuum pump. One is that it doesn't have to be purchased with a prescription. If you are shy about discussing your ED issues with your health care team, you can purchase this tool with or without their knowledge. It is relatively inexpensive when compared to other ED treatments, but most insurance plans, including Medicare, cover it when it is purchased with a doctor's prescription.

As with the constriction ring, the vacuum pump also restricts the flow of blood, may cause the penis to be wobbly at the base, and can turn it a bluish color that is cold to the touch. Unlike the constriction ring, the vacuum pump adds a pumping action that can cause some bruising, discomfort, or pain. The constriction ring that accompanies the pump must be removed within 30 minutes.

Statistics show that all men are able achieve some level of success with a vacuum pump. If you try this option, learn how to use it properly and give yourself plenty of time to perfect your technique.

Practice Makes Perfect

"The pump takes time and patience, but you can get really good at this if you practice using it. I found it awkward at first, but I refused to give up and finally got the hang of it. It was worth it. This is a great, drug-free treatment."—*Doug*

Penile support sleeve

The penile support sleeve is a unique item that enables you to have intercourse without an erection. It is easy to use and is ideal for men who are uncomfortable with other treatment choices or have physical issues that prevent them from achieving an erection. The sleeve is available at online and retail stores, comes in different sizes, and will not interfere with the natural development of an erection if one takes place. It is also disposable.

Even if you have severe chronic disease or physical issues that have prevented you from engaging in intercourse, you can use the sleeve.

When using this product, generously lubricate the sleeve and hold the penis securely at its base. You may find that certain sexual positions are

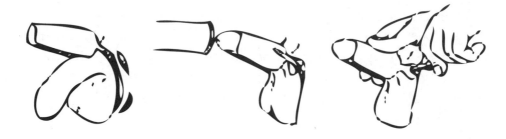

more comfortable than others. If you have your partner take the upper position during intimate activity, the sleeve-covered penis may be easier to use.

Another Chance for Intimacy

Phillip has type 2 diabetes and has multiple physical complications. He uses a wheelchair to get around because his left leg was amputated several years ago. He just learned that he needs an additional amputation. He has kidney failure and must have dialysis several times each week. He is also blind in one eye. He may have lost a lot, but he hasn't lost his true love, his wife, Alice. The two of them had a single request that they brought to his diabetes educator—to enjoy physical intimacy one more time.

When his educator suggested that he try a penile sleeve, he was initially unconvinced. How could it be a pleasurable experience? But it was. It was a bit awkward to secure in place at first, but it stayed on with the help of a condom that he placed over it. For the first time in many years, Phillip and Alice connected in a physical way that matched their emotional connection. Both were extremely grateful for the ability to do this.

Implants

A penile implant is surgically placed into the penis and creates a natural-looking erection. There are several different models available, but the most common and effective is the three-piece inflatable one. It consists of two cylinders that are placed in the penis, a pump to inflate and deflate it, which is placed into the scrotum next to the testicles, and a reservoir of fluid that is placed into the abdomen.

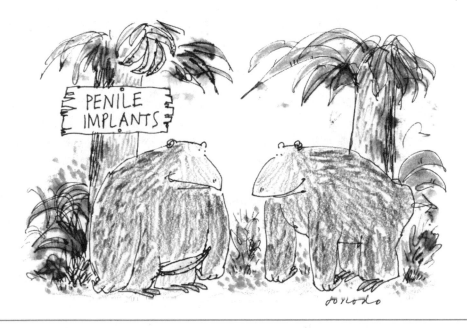

When you squeeze the pump, it transfers the fluid from the reservoir to the cylinders and creates an erection. The penis can stay erect all day without harm and lovemaking can be prolonged until your partner is satisfied. As with any mechanical device, it may eventually need to be replaced. Another type is made of a flexible stick that you bend down during regular activity and straighten out when you participate in intimacy. Both are pictured below.

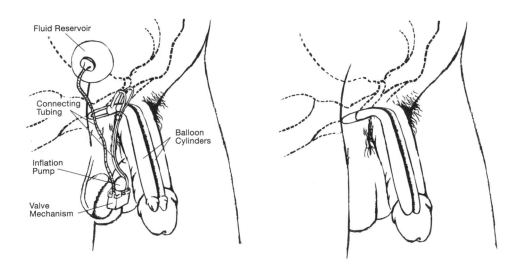

Impact and Ease of Implant

"The surgery was done under general anesthesia, which wasn't a problem for me. Depending on the technique that your doctor uses, it could be done as an inpatient or outpatient. Unlike the other tools, I don't have to carry anything around with me and I always have a natural looking and feeling erection. I love my implant. I tell everyone that it was the best thing that I ever did for myself." —*Frank*

Counseling

You may not like to share your feelings, but for many men, the psychological component of ED responds well to professional emotional support. A qualified mental health counselor can help you determine if your problem is due to stress, relationship issues, self-imposed performance pressure, or a physical problem that requires medical attention. Visit *www.AASECT.org*, the official website of the American Association of Sex Educators, Counselors, and Therapists to find a qualified therapist.

Constructive Counseling

"Our therapist helped me put my diabetes issues into perspective and helped Kim learn to support me in a more constructive way. Our sessions made a huge difference in our relationship, and our sex life is back on track." —*Phillip*

As you have learned, there are numerous treatment options and one size does not fit all. You should be able to find an option that works well for you and your partner. Don't give up! As you can see, there are many treatments available to treat ED. Discuss these options with your partner and choose one that works best for your particular needs. Meet with your physician and ask him or her to provide you with the product and education needed to use it successfully.

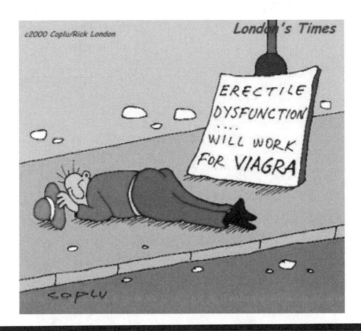

FOR YOU AND YOUR PARTNER

1 Which treatment options are you and your partner willing to try?

2 Which option do you feel will bring you both closest to your desired sexual outcome?

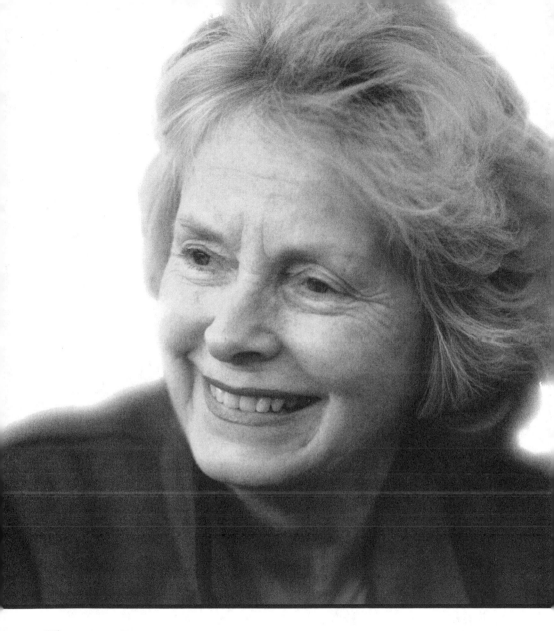

Chapter 5
For Her

In this chapter:
- Learn about sexual complications.
- Explore a variety of treatment options.

REMEMBER THE MOVIE *When Harry Met Sally*, starring Billy Crystal and Meg Ryan? There is a famous scene in a restaurant in which Sally tries to convince Harry that "most women, at one time or another, have faked it (orgasm)." Harry claims that he has never been fooled.

Sally: "Oh right. That's right. I forgot. You're a man."
Harry: "What is that supposed to mean?"
Sally: "Nothing. It's just that all men are sure it never happens to them, and most women at one time or another have done it, so you do the math."
Harry: "You don't think that I can tell the difference?"
Sally: "No."
Harry: "Get outta here."

Many jokes have been made about women who pretend to achieve sexual satisfaction. Whether they are true or not, these jokes highlight an important reality—many women do not fully enjoy intimate activity with their partners. Back in 1995, Ann Landers, the well-known advice columnist, asked women if they preferred to be held close or participate in sexual intercourse. Seventy-two percent of the women said that they preferred to be held. If you and your partner are satisfied with how you interact in the bedroom, that's great. If you are unhappy, your problems may be related to your diabetes.

DIABETES-RELATED SEXUAL COMPLICATIONS

For years, most experts ignored the possibility of diabetes-related sexual complications in women. Fortunately, studies are now ongoing, so we are learning more about this important area. While there are numerous non-diabetes-related stresses that can create intimacy challenges for a woman—such as hormonal swings, and family and work pressures—diabetes can be a cause as well. Sex-related complications can affect a woman's ability to enjoy a rich and fulfilling intimate and emotional relationship.

So far, we've discussed ways that diabetes can affect both men and women and their intimate relationships. As a woman, however, you may have diabetes-related symptoms that affect you in a unique way. Let's review some of these needs and talk about ways to deal with them.

Problem: Your blood sugar level interferes with intimate activity

Blood Sugar Lows Can Interrupt Intimacy

"Sam and I were enjoying our first weekend away in a long time. Between our jobs and kids, we rarely have time for each other. This getaway was just what the doctor ordered. Our evening started with a lovely dinner in the hotel restaurant and several glasses of wine. We even danced a bit, which was a real treat! After that, we took a lovely walk on the beach then headed back to our room. Just as we were getting intimate, my blood sugar level dropped. I tested after dinner and thought that all was well, but it wasn't. As my level plunged, I stopped responding to anything that Sam said or did. Fortunately, he recognized the symptoms and grabbed a can of juice from the room's mini-bar. I responded quickly to the juice, but was left with an enormous headache. We were both so disappointed. I was no longer in the mood, so Sam went out for a walk."—*Nina*

Abnormal blood glucose levels can stop a lovely evening of intimate activity right in its tracks. Here are some ways to keep this situation from happening to you:

Check your blood sugar level prior to sexual activity

It may remove some of the spontaneity of the moment, but will help prevent an unexpected hypoglycemic event from occurring at an inopportune moment. Sexual activity is exercise and you should prepare for it in the same way that you prepare for any other workout. If you inject insulin, adjust your dose the way you would for any physical workout. If you wear a pump, switch to your temporary exercise basal rate or disconnect altogether. Test before and after and treat abnormal blood sugar levels as needed. Keep fast-acting glucose snacks nearby. Nina was lucky to find some juice in her hotel room's fridge. If there had been no fast-acting snack nearby, her mild hypoglycemic event could have become far more serious.

Limit your alcohol intake

Alcohol is permitted on most diabetic meal plans, but can cause your blood sugar level to drop rapidly, especially if you don't eat any food with it. The American Diabetes Association recommends that women limit their intake to one drink (or less per day, and two drinks or less per day for an adult male).

A drink is defined as:
- 12 oz of beer
- 5 oz of wine
- 1.5 oz distilled spirits

Be sure to enjoy your alcoholic beverage with a complete meal or small snack, which will help limit the blood sugar–lowering effect of the alcohol. If you have a history of alcohol problems, you should not indulge in alcohol at all.

Monitor your blood sugar when you eat out

When you cook at home, you know exactly what goes into each recipe. When you eat out, you may ingest an unexpected ingredient that changes your glucose level or your insulin need. Ask your waiter about the dishes that you wish to order.

Note your "time of the month"

If you have diabetes, your blood sugar level may be sensitive to your menstrual cycle. Some women experience blood sugar increases while others drop during this time. Be aware that a low may occur during any type of affectionate activity.

Test more frequently if you are menopausal

Blood sugar levels tend to be more unpredictable as a woman enters menopause. This is due to the hormonal irregularities that exist during this time. Prepare for the unexpected and keep appropriate snacks handy.

Remember yesterday's workout

A single day of physical activity can help lower your blood glucose level for the next several days. If you worked out yesterday and plan to be sexually active this evening, the combined blood glucose–lowering effect of your workout plus your evening actions may cause a rapid drop in blood sugar. Again, test frequently and snack as needed.

Problem: The thrill is gone

In chapter 2, we reviewed many emotional issues that affect libido. If no obvious emotional reason exists, the problem may be a physical one. If your hormone levels are not within a normal range, your depression medication has stopped working, or your blood sugar level is abnormal, you will probably feel less interest in being sexual.

Ask your doctor about hormone treatments

Testosterone is a natural male hormone that is also produced in certain levels in women. Some physicians use it to help women with diabetes regain their libido. Testosterone dosing must be carefully determined and tracked, as these levels can quickly climb. High levels of testosterone in women can lead to excess facial hair, male-type hair loss, and acne, among other things.

Ask your health care team about Viagra

Viagra and other similar medications are no longer the exclusive domain of men. These drugs have helped many women with their libido issues. Discuss this option with your physician.

Improve your blood sugar control

If your blood sugar level is difficult to control, discuss different medication options with your health care team. As we mentioned earlier, there are many oral medications, injected medicines, such as Byetta and Symlin, and different insulin options to choose from. Many women have enjoyed enhanced control with the use of an insulin pump.

Choose another antidepressant

Some antidepressants known as selective serotonin reuptake inhibitors (SSRIs), which include Prozac, Paxil, and Zoloft, can cause a drop in your libido. These medications cause a drop in dopamine, which is a chemical in the brain that helps you enjoy pleasurable experiences. If you use an SSRI and have noticed a change in your sexual interest, the following medications may help relieve this problem:

- bupropion
- buspirone
- methylphenidate
- mirtazapine
- amphetamine
- pramipexole
- ropinirole

Some antidepressant medications, such as Wellbutrin SR, Serzone, Remeron, and Lovox are less likely to cause sexual problems.

Problem: You are too tired

Abnormal blood glucose levels will tire you out. They can happen for a variety of reasons, including your food choices and medication use. You may also experience a significant amount of fatigue while you recover from a low blood sugar episode. While you feel this way, the last thing on your mind is how to be a vixen in the bedroom.

Diabetes Causing Exhaustion

"Sid used to tease me when I said that I was too tired for 'fun.' Well it's happening so often now that it isn't humorous any longer. Some days, I can barely make it through dinner. I don't know what it is. I have had type 2 diabetes for about four years and have never felt this exhausted before. I have to do something about this."—*Stacy*

Don't follow fad diets

An extremely low-carbohydrate meal plan can leave you feeling tired. Carbohydrate-containing foods such as rice, breads, pasta, fruit, fruit juices, milk, yogurt, and starchy vegetables give your body the type of energy that it needs. The American Diabetes Association and other recognized health organizations recommend that your intake of carbohydrates be 45–65% of your total calories and not less than 130 grams of carbohydrates per day. Meet with a registered dietitian to help you determine the amount that is right for you.

Don't limit your calories too severely

It is tempting to cut your food intake drastically to help lose unwanted weight quickly. This practice is unhealthy, can cause you to feel lethargic, and puts you at risk for developing serious medical problems. The key to healthy weight loss is food portion control and regular physical activity. There are some medications that have come on the market that help individuals with diabetes lose extra pounds. Several helpful weight loss suggestions are highlighted in chapter 3.

Don't skip meals

When you go longer than five hours without a meal or snack, your blood glucose level can drop and you will feel tired. If your schedule doesn't allow you to sit down for a meal, keep diabetes-friendly snacks, such as nuts, crackers, and dried fruit in your purse or car. Several diabetes companies make snack bars and meal replacement shakes, which are also handy to carry.

Exercise

Physical activity releases endorphins that raise your spirit and help you feel energized. Choose an activity that you enjoy or enlist a friend to do it with you. Sex is a form of exercise and is a healthy and fun way to keep your heart strong, spirits high, and relationships healthy.

Keep your blood sugar level within a healthy range

Think about the last time you treated a blood glucose low. Most people feel unwell for several hours following a hypoglycemic event. Check your blood glucose level often and treat any low levels using the 15/15 Rule, as explained in chapter 3, or as directed by your health care team.

Get plenty of rest

For most busy women, this is almost impossible to do. Your body needs rest. If you have difficulty falling asleep, examine the hours leading up to bedtime.

Helpful Tips for Falling Asleep

1. Avoid caffeine close to bedtime. Many people find it helpful to switch to caffeine-free beverages after lunchtime.
2. Turn off the outside world before you head to bed. If you watch the news right before retiring or fall asleep with the television on, the events highlighted on the news can keep you awake or disturb your sleep.
3. Keep a pen and notepad by your bed to jot down thoughts that pop into your head as you fall asleep. It is hard to relax when you are struggling to keep in mind thoughts you will need to remember for the following day.
4. Don't rely on alcohol as a sleep aid. A glass of wine may help you fall asleep initially, but it can disturb your sleep during the night. Research shows that alcohol interrupts natural sleep cycles. An alcohol-induced sleep is not a relaxing one.
5. Review the stress-lowering suggestions highlighted in chapter 2.

Explore other ways to be intimate

Sexual activity doesn't always have to lead to intercourse. Watch television together and cuddle. Enjoy each other's presence. Take a walk and hold hands. Use this time as an investment in your relationship. You may be too tired to engage in more involved physical activity, but you can still communicate in a loving way.

Arrange for household help

Many women believe that they can "do it all," but few can. It is exhausting to try to balance a career and a family life. Try the following:

- Have a housekeeper come into your home to assist you with the heavy cleaning.
- Have your weekly grocery order delivered.
- Use the Internet to order personal care items and household goods, such as shampoo, hand cream, kitchenware, etc.

Don't let diabetes overwhelm you

Use the Jump Start Pledge technique mentioned in chapter 2 to help add new diabetes care tasks to your life in a gentle way.

Problem: You have trouble lubricating

Without adequate vaginal lubrication, intercourse can be unpleasant or even painful. The nerves that tell the body to release lubricant into the vaginal area can become damaged if your blood sugar levels stay elevated over an extended period of time, such as a few months or several years.

Sudden Problems with Lubrication

"Kevin and I have been married for three years and never had a problem before. I just don't understand. I'm only 28, way too young for menopause, right? So, why won't my body lubricate anymore when I am still so sexually turned on by my husband?" —*Amy*

Use a water-based lubricant

Today, there are many effective water-based lubricants on the market that can replace the lubrication you lack. Any brand that is made specifically for the vaginal area will work. If you plan to become pregnant, however, review your lubricant choice with your obstetrician. Certain brands may damage sperm and reduce your ability to conceive.

Maintain your blood sugar level within a healthy target range

Use all of the suggestions highlighted throughout this book to bring your level into a range that has been suggested by your health care team.

Allow plenty of time for touching, caressing, and romance

If your sexual activity is rushed, your body may not have time to become aroused.

Ask your physician about hormones

In certain post-menopausal women, estrogen supplementation can help reduce vaginal dryness and improve tactile sensation in the pelvic area by improving blood flow and the quality of the vaginal lining.

Teach your body through touch

Masturbation can help train your body to lubricate when stimulated.

Problem: You can no longer achieve an orgasm

If you have diabetes-related damage to certain nerves in the body, you may lose the ability to have an orgasm or need a higher level of stimulation and additional time to do so.

Normalize your blood sugar level

This has been highlighted several times throughout this chapter. The advice holds true for this situation as well.

Maintain a healthy blood pressure level

Healthy blood circulation is important for a woman's sexual performance. If your body is unable to send an adequate amount of blood flow to the pelvic region, you will have a difficult time becoming aroused. Healthy blood pressure also protects your kidneys and enables your body to function properly. Treatments for lowering your blood pressure include:

- medication
- stress-reduction activities
- regular physical activity
- sodium restriction

Take your time

As mentioned earlier, a women's libido is on a slow simmer that gradually develops into a greater amount of passion.

"The basic conflict between men and women, sexually, is that men are like firemen and women are like fire. To men, sex is an emergency, and no matter what [they're] doing, [they] can be ready in two minutes. Women, on the other hand, are like fire. They're very exciting, but the conditions have to be exactly right for it to occur." —*Jerry Seinfeld*

If you need more romance, cuddling, and foreplay in order to get into the mood, arrange for it to happen. Send the kids to sleep over at a friend or relative's house and create an atmosphere that relaxes you and helps put you into the mood for sexual activity. Go away for a night or a weekend with your spouse. Create moments that enable you and your partner to relax and enjoy each other.

Communicate with your partner

If he wants to share his loving touch with you and you are unable to reach a climax, he may believe that he has failed to meet your needs. Let him know that this is caused by your diabetes. That information should help remove guilt or ill feelings from the bedroom.

Experiment with a greater variety of foreplay techniques

Oral stimulation by your partner may help you become more aroused prior to vaginal intercourse. Speak with your partner and try new techniques together.

Practice

When you are by yourself, experiment with different masturbation techniques. You may discover new ways to become aroused and can teach your partner to incorporate them into your lovemaking.

Problem: You've developed skin problems

Intimacy can involve touching. Poor diabetes control can cause a person to develop a variety of different skin changes that make a loving touch more difficult to enjoy. If the nerves that go to different parts of the body become damaged, that area may lose its ability to sweat properly. If this occurs, your hands and feet may become extremely dry and crack, while your face and trunk may sweat excessively. Dry skin can also develop if your blood sugar level runs high, which can prompt you to urinate more frequently. As you run to the bathroom, you lose fluid and become more dehydrated.

Pain Preventing Intimacy

"We used to hold hands, but my skin has become so dry that I don't want George to hold them anymore. I've used every cream that I can find, including the ones made especially for people with diabetes, but nothing helps. I know that handholding is not a huge deal, but I really miss it."—*Sharon*

Maintain your blood sugar level in a healthy range

This suggestion has been made repeatedly because it can make a difference in so many areas.

Limit or avoid certain foods that trigger sweating

These include chocolate, red wine, cheese, some sodas, and spicy foods. Each person is unique. Certain foods may cause you to sweat, while others won't. Observe your body's reaction to the foods in this list and avoid or limit those that affect you.

Stay hydrated

Most individuals meet their hydration needs if they drink when they feel thirsty. Your needs may be different, especially if you have other medical issues, such as kidney disease. Speak with your health care team about the amount of fluid that you should consume.

For dry skin, use creams and oils to lubricate your skin

Avoid creams that contain alcohol, which can dry your skin and cause it to crack. If you put cream onto your feet, avoid the area between your toes. This area tends to stay moist, which can invite harmful bacteria to grow.

Problem: You have frequent urinary tract infections

Frustration Over Persistent Problem

"'Come on, not again.' That's what Randy said last night when I told him that I had another yeast infection. I'm getting so tired of these and poor Randy has lost his patience. Now we have to take the medication and hope that it won't return. I don't know what to do anymore. We are both sick of this."—*Nancy*

A poorly timed yeast or bladder infection can ruin a night of romance. Women who have diabetes tend to develop more urinary tract infections than those without the disease. If your blood sugar level is not well controlled, bacteria will flourish in the highly sweet environment. Common symptoms of yeast infections include:

- vaginal itching
- irritated skin in the vaginal area
- burning or pain during intercourse
- pain while urinating
- white vaginal discharge that resembles cottage cheese

Symptoms of a bladder infection may include:

- a frequent urge to urinate
- a heavy feeling in the lower abdomen
- unpleasant-smelling urine
- pain beneath your rib cage

There are numerous yeast infection treatments on the market today, but you should see a physician to correctly identify the problem. Bladder infections require prescription medication. Here are some ways to help prevent these problems from occurring.

Empty your bladder regularly

Urinate immediately after you engage in sexual intercourse.

Don't introduce bacteria into the vaginal area

After using the toilet, wipe from front to back to avoid bringing bacteria into the vaginal area. Bathe regularly and make sure that you and your partner are clean prior to engaging in sexual intercourse.

Stay hydrated

Drink a generous amount of water each day—at least eight glasses should be your goal.

Increase your intake of Lactobacillus organisms

Drink acidophilus milk or eat low-fat, artificially sweetened, or plain yogurt that contains live Lactobacillus organisms. It can help you maintain a normal balance of organisms in the vaginal area.

Wear cotton underwear

This helps prevent moisture from accumulating in the vaginal area.

Avoid tight-fitting clothing

They increase your body heat and encourage moisture to develop in the vaginal area.

Avoid perfumes in the vaginal area

Do not use scented toilet paper, deodorant tampons, perfumes, or feminine sprays. Avoid douching. These products alter the delicate balance of organisms in your vaginal area.

Limit your use of antibiotics

Don't take them unless they are absolutely necessary. They can alter your normal balance of vaginal organisms and encourage the overgrowth of yeast. If you must use antibiotics take a probiotic (Lactobacillus capsule) before and during your antibiotic treatment to reduce this effect. Probiotic products can be purchased at a local health food store. If you continue to develop urinary tract infections after sexual intercourse, ask your physician if you should take antibiotics after intercourse or on a regular basis.

Drink artificially sweetened cranberry juice

This is helpful if you develop a bladder infection. Be sure to include the additional carbohydrate amount in your meal plan.

Choose your form of contraceptive carefully

If you develop repeat infections, use a form of contraception other than a diaphragm and/or spermicidal jelly.

Problem: You are afraid of getting pregnant

If you are worried about becoming pregnant, you will probably find it more difficult to relax during intimacy. That concern can make intercourse painful and distance you from the rich bonding experience that should happen during intimate moments. It is important to achieve

Fear of Pregnancy with Diabetes

Tammy and Jack have decided to have a baby. Tammy has diabetes and knows that she must get her A1C level within a healthy range before she conceives. Unfortunately, her last A1C was 9%, which is not a healthy level for her or for anyone who wishes to become pregnant. Because her diabetes control is not optimal yet and she doesn't trust her birth control to protect her, she is nervous about being intimate with her husband, Jack. Jack thinks that her attitude has gotten out of hand. He understands that she must lower her A1C, but why does he have to be punished? He doesn't like being rejected and is tired of living the celibate life. His wife's new fear is making life very difficult for both of them.

excellent diabetes control for several months before you become pregnant. Both you and your partner may also worry that your children may develop diabetes; that concern can bring stress into your bedroom as well.

Choose a reliable birth control

Have your OBGYN help you and your partner choose a contraceptive method or combination of methods that fit your lifestyle. Become comfortable with it and use it each and every time you engage in sexual activity. Oral contraceptives that contain a combination of estrogen and progestin (or are sequential) are associated with a variety of heart problems and complications. Pills that contain less than 35 mg estrogen are generally recommended. Pills that contain progestin alone may increase lipid and glucose levels.

The Norplant System is a form of contraceptive that may cause menstrual irregularities, an increase in lipids, and glucose resistance. If you choose to use this, you may need to increase your insulin dose. Progesterone containing intrauterine devices may cause pain, irregular bleeding, perforation of the uterus, and infection. Any type of injury can cause blood sugar levels to climb. Other devices, including the diaphragm, condoms, and cervical caps should not affect your diabetes control.

Learn about family risk factors

You may also worry that your baby will develop diabetes. Diabetes is indeed a disease with a genetic link, and your chances of contracting it increases if members of your immediate family have already been diagnosed.

Share the discussion about expanding your family with your partner. If you agree that it is time to attempt a pregnancy, work together with your OBGYN and other members of your health care team to prepare for pregnancy.

Don't allow your diabetes to interfere with your ability to physically connect with your sexual partner. Discuss problems that you are having with your health care team and your loved one. Each woman's diabetes experience is different and so is her sexual relationship. Work with your health care team to find a solution that will work for both of you.

Chances of Developing Diabetes

Family Member with Diabetes	Chance Child Will Develop Diabetes
No Diabetes in the Family	11% chance of type 2 diabetes by age 70 1% chance of type 1 diabetes by age 50
*One Parent with Type 1 Diabetes*** Father with type 1 diabetes	6% chance of type 1 diabetes
Mother with type 1 diabetes who was younger than 25 when the child was born	4% chance of type 1 diabetes
Mother with type 1 diabetes who was older than 25 when the child was born	1% chance of type 1 diabetes
One Parent with Type 2 Diabetes Diagnosed before the age of 50	14% chance of type 2 diabetes
Both Parents with Type 2 Diabetes Overall risk	45% chance of type 2 diabetes by age 65

** Risk doubles if the parent was diagnosed by the age of 11

101 Tips for a Healthy Pregnancy with Diabetes (American Diabetes Association)

FOR YOU AND YOUR PARTNER

1 What type of women's issues has diabetes brought to your life?

2 How can you and your partner support each other when these occur?

3 If you are planning to become pregnant, what can you both do to prepare for this?

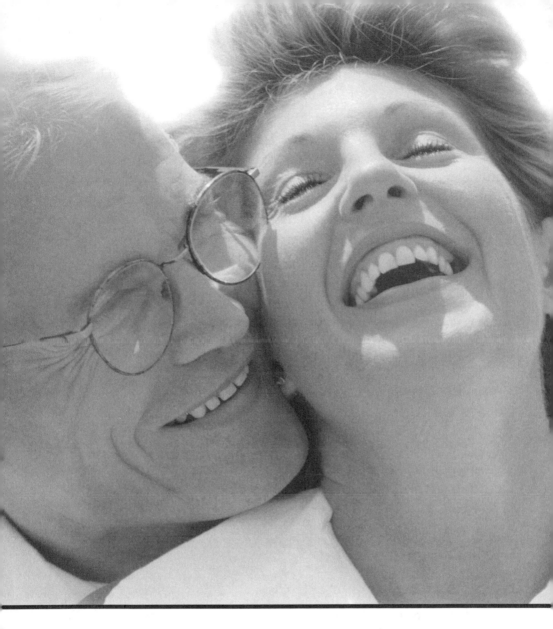

Chapter 6
For Fun

In this chapter:

- Learn additional ways to enhance your intimate relationships.
- Find out about aphrodisiacs that can enhance your sexual experience.
- Discover the possible value of herbal supplements.

IF YOU ARE STRUGGLING with sexual complications, interactions with your partner are probably filled with tension and discomfort. Relax and enjoy your love life once again through sensual touching, massage, aphrodisiacs, and other great options.

We've discussed pills, creams, injections, and suppositories. These help return a level of normalcy to the act of intercourse, but sexual intimacy is far more than that. At its best, it is an interaction that brings joy and fulfillment to two individuals who choose to be together. The following can help you rekindle sensuous feelings.

SENSUAL TOUCHING

Relaxing Techniques

Suzette recently began using a vaginal lubricant to reduce her discomfort during sexual activity. It works fine, but the memories of past painful episodes are still fresh in her mind and cause her to tense up whenever her husband suggests a night of romance. To help her relax and get in the mood once again, she and her husband used a technique called sensual touching. They loved the results. It brought a new dimension to their lovemaking that both she and her husband appreciated greatly, especially after 12 years of marriage.

The sexual touching technique can help you relax, connect with your partner, and explore areas of your body that respond to intimate touch. When diabetes enters the bedroom, it often introduces stress and anxiety into this important area of your life. This technique can help you overcome that. Try it at a time when you won't be rushed. While disrobed to whatever degree is comfortable for you, take turns touching each other with a variety of soft objects—a feather, blush applicator, silk scarf, etc. Visit sensitive areas that you may have never paid attention to before.

- the hairline
- eyebrows
- forehead
- eyelids
- temple
- cheeks

The ultimate goal is to enjoy a new level of intimate communication and knowledge about each other. It can be followed by intercourse or used by itself, which can remove a great deal of performance anxiety.

KISSING

Before the birth control pill arrived on the scene in the 1960s, "making out," physical pleasure without intercourse, was a popular way for couples to interact. When you remove the pressure to complete the act and just take things slowly, you will open up a world that you may not have realized existed before. There is no need to focus on intercourse as the ultimate goal of intimate activity. Take it slow. The slower you move, the more sexual tension you can create. That should help both of you relax and improve your sexual response. It can also take the pressure off of either of you to perform. Turn back the clock to simpler times.

NEW POSITIONS AND NEW LOCATIONS

Introducing a new sexual position to your lovemaking can heighten the excitement. You can learn new approaches to intimacy by viewing movies or reading books on the subject. If you have developed any physical ailments that interfere with the position that you are accustomed to using, a new way to approach intercourse may enable you to reconnect with your partner again. Changing the location of your lovemaking can also heighten the excitement. If possible, take a mini vacation to a hotel or just try a different location in your own home.

SURPRISE ONE ANOTHER

You and your partner may respond positively to an unexpected romantic gesture. It could be a surprise candlelit dinner, a loving text message, or a sugarless candy hidden in a briefcase. When you feel wanted by your mate, your desire to be together can be enhanced.

SHARE SEXUAL SECRETS

Let your partner know how you enjoy being touched. Many couples keep quiet and don't get their physical needs addressed.

EXPLORE EROTIC MEDIA

Spice up your love life, learn new techniques, and encourage your body to respond more enthusiastically by sharing erotic media, such as DVDs, films, books, and magazines with your loved one. These products are available throughout the Internet and by mail order. If you feel uncomfortable about having these items in your home, consider viewing one of today's many sexually charged R-rated films. They can be rented, without any embarrassment, from your local video store.

R-rated Films

9½ Weeks	Dangerous Beauty
"10"	Eyes Wide Shut
American Beauty	Monster's Ball
American Gigolo	Sex, Lies, and Videotape
An Officer and a Gentleman	Showgirls
Basic Instinct	Striptease
Body Heat	Unfaithful
Boogie Nights	Wild Things

ABSTAIN

Most people desire what they can't have. Orthodox Jews have a very interesting approach to sexuality. For two weeks out of the month, a married couple will physically stay apart. They can't touch, hug, or even kiss. During that time, sexual tension begins to build. When the two weeks are over, the woman immerses herself in a ritual bath and their physical relationship begins anew. Many couples who have been married for decades continue to enjoy a honeymoon-like reconnection with their spouse each month. If your love life has become routine or has been filled with performance tension, schedule a mini sexual vacation. Give yourselves time to yearn for each other.

MASSAGE

Alternatives to Medication

David has type 2 diabetes and recently developed erectile dysfunction. He has successful sexual relations with his wife when he takes Levitra or uses a vacuum pump, but doesn't always want to plan ahead for sexual activity. Sometimes he just wants to do something spontaneous. So he and his wife Charlotte found that massage helped them experience closeness without performance pressure. "We purchased an instructional video and did our best to learn the techniques. We aren't great at it, but have lots of fun."

The muscle kneading action and smooth flowing motions of massage can improve circulation, relax muscle tension, and feel great. You don't have to be a professionally trained masseuse to add this tool to your intimate repertoire. Create your own style and let feedback from your partner guide your movement. He or she can tell you what feels good and what doesn't. If you hit a ticklish area, laugh together and enjoy the effort. If you want to heighten the experience, take a class, read a book, or visit an instructional website such as *www.massagefree.com* that offers direction from a professional therapist.

Like sensual touching, massage offers you and your partner an opportunity to give and receive physical pleasure. There are numerous types of nonsexual massage that exist.

▮ Swedish
▮ reflexology
▮ shiatsu
▮ acupressure
▮ aromatherapy

Adding Romance Through Massage

"It's a new hobby. Instead of complaining about how much diabetes was stealing from our nights, we began to explore new ways to relax and enjoy our time together."—*Tom and Nina*

Fran especially enjoyed having her husband massage her feet. As a person with diabetes, they have always been a source of worry. Caressing them has helped her feel less nervous about their health.

Relieving the Stress of Diabetes

"I'm terrified of amputation. My friend had so much trouble with her feet because of her diabetes that she had to have two toes amputated. I check my feet every day, visit a podiatrist often, and never walk around barefoot. My feet really make me nervous." When her husband Carl began massaging the soles of her feet, she experienced a tremendous feeling of relief. "These were my frightening feet and they were getting superstar treatment! I couldn't thank Carl enough. What a relaxing and wonderful gift."—*Fran*

Enhance any massage by using scented essential oils. These natural oils are sold in health food stores. Here are several popular scents along with the effect that they can have on your moods.

Suggested Ways
to Use Aromatherapy Oils

1. Add scent to a room. Place 2–3 drops into a spray bottle filled with water. Spray into the air as desired.

2. Enhance a cozy evening with a favorite aroma. Place several drops into the wax as a candle burns. If you use your fireplace, place 2–3 drops of atlas cedarwood, cypress, frankincense, myrrh, or vetivert, onto a dried log. Let the oil soak in before adding the log to the fire.

3. Keep the bathroom fresh. Put a drop of oil onto several cotton balls and place them throughout the room.

4. Remove some stress from your office. Place a drop onto a light bulb. When the lamp is turned on, the bulb's warmth will release the scent into the room.

5. Have sweet dreams. Add one or two drops to a washcloth and toss it into the dryer to scent your towels and sheets.

6. Perfume your lingerie. When hand washing delicates, add a drop of oil to the rinse water.

7. Create a signature perfume. Add 25 drops of your favorite scent to 1 ounce of perfume alcohol. Let it sit for two weeks before use.

8. Help relieve a headache. Combine 1 drop of peppermint oil with 1 teaspoon of vegetable oil. Rub onto the back of your neck.

9. Prepare scented massage oil. Combine 3 to 5 drops with an ounce of Jojoba oil or other skin-friendly oil.

Aromatherapy Massage Oils

Basil—energizing, invigorating, and refreshing
Chamomile—relaxing, soothes aches and itchy skin
Cinnamon—stimulating, uplifting
Clary Sage—arousing, invigorating, gently erotic, and uplifting
Eucalyptus—relaxing and for muscle aches, colds, and flu
Frankincense—rejuvenating, soothing, relaxing
Geranium—puts you to sleep or puts you in a good mood
Jasmine—erotic, exotic, and soothing
Juniper—boosts energy and reduces stress (do not use during pregnancy)
Lavender—stimulant and sedative, calming, refreshing, restoring
Lemon—wakes up the mind and body, stimulating, arousing
Neroli—hypnotically soothing, good for tension and anxiety
Patchouli—stimulating, erotic, arousing
Peppermint—invigorates, refreshes, warms, and energizes
Rose—seductive, romantic, soothing, and calming
Rosemary—energizing, invigorating, and clears the head
Sandalwood—heady, sensual, deeply soothing
Tea-tree—healing, calming, good for aches, abrasions, and fungal infections
Thyme—uplifting, invigorating stimulant, good for stress or anxiety
Ylang-ylang—sensual, seductive, deeply relaxing

EXERCISE

Everyone, especially a person with diabetes, benefits from regular physical activity. Share your workout with your partner. Sharing time at the gym can wake up other areas of your body and heighten your sexual interest in each other. Here are some exercises and suggested activities that you might enjoy doing with your spouse or partner along with the amount of calories that they use.

Activity Calorie Calculator

Light Activity	Calories/hour	Calories/minute
Strolling, 1.0 mile/hour	150	2.5
Golf, using power cart	175	3.0
Level walking, 2.0 miles/hour	200	3.5

Moderate Activity	Calories/hour	Calories/minute
Cycling, 5.5 miles/hour	210	3.5
Gardening	220	3.5
Canoeing, 2.5 miles/hour	230	4.0
Walking, 3.0 miles/hour	275	4.5
Bowling	300	5.0
Golf, pulling cart	300	5.0
Row boating, 2.5 miles/hour	300	5.0
Swimming, 0.25 miles/hour	300	5.0
Cycling, 8 miles/hour	325	5.5
Golf, carrying clubs	350	6.0
Badminton	350	6.0
Horseback riding, trotting	350	6.0
Square dancing	350	6.0
Volleyball	350	6.0
Roller skating	350	6.0
Doubles tennis	360	6.0
Table tennis	360	6.0
Walking, 4.0 miles/hour	360	6.0

Strenuous Activity	Calories/hour	Calories/minute
Vigorous dancing	320–500	5.5–8.5
Cycling, 10 miles/hour	400	6.5
Ice skating, 10 miles/hour	400	6.5
Walking, 5 miles/hour	420	7.0
Cycling, 11 miles/hour	420	7.0
Singles tennis	420	7.0
Waterskiing	480	8.0

(continued on page 98)

Activity Calorie Calculator (continued from page 97)

Strenuous Activity	Calories/hour	Calories/minute
Jogging, 5 miles/hour	480	8.0
Cycling, 12 miles/hour	480	8.0
Hill climbing, 100 feet/hour	490	8.0
Downhill skiing	550	9.0
Running, 5.5 miles/hour	600	10.0
Squash and handball	600	11.0
Cycling, 13 miles/hour	660	11.0
Running, 6–9 miles/hour	660–850	11.0–14.0
Cross-country skiing	600–1,200	10.0–20.0
Running, 10 miles/hour	900	15.0

Life with Diabetes, 3rd Edition (American Diabetes Association)

Sexual Activity Calorie Burning

As we've mentioned previously, sexual activity also counts as physical activity. Here are the calories that are burned:

Level of sexual activity	Calories/ 15 minutes	Calories/hour
Active, with vigorous effort	9	34
General activity, moderate effort	5	20
Passive activity, light effort, kissing, hugging	0	0

www.calorielab.com, 2007

Set up a workout schedule with your partner. If you are walkers, challenge each other to meet a daily step total goal. You can do this by buying his and hers pedometers.

1. Wear your pedometer every day for a single week. Don't alter your physical activity level at all. Just go about your business as usual.
2. At the end of the week, determine the average number of steps that you take each day.
3. Add 1,000 steps/day to that total. This is your new daily goal.
4. Challenge your partner to meet his or her goal.

Ways to meet your walking goals

▌ Take the stairs instead of the elevator
▌ Park your car at the back of the lot and walk to your destination
▌ Pace while talking on the phone
▌ Go for a walk
▌ Walk over to a co-worker's office instead of calling or emailing them
▌ Walk during work breaks
▌ When shopping, push your cart up and down all of the aisles

APHRODISIACS

"When you come down to it, the power of the human mind is probably the most potent aphrodisiac of all."—*Varro E. Tyler, PhD, ScD*

Since ancient times, man has searched for foods and scents that increase sexual interest and potency. Some claim that aphrodisiac foods contain active ingredients that heighten sexual responses, but other experts believe that they trigger what is known as a placebo effect. This is the trick that our mind plays on our body when we use products that have little or no value. If we believe that an item works, we may experience an actual benefit.

Placebos contain harmless, ineffective ingredients and are frequently used in research to test the effectiveness of new medications. One group of subjects will take a dose of medication, while another group will use a placebo. If the medicine out performs the placebo, it is considered effective.

The following are several aphrodisiac foods that have been singled out throughout history because of their active ingredients, or their

Foods That May Contain Active Sexually Enhancing Ingredients

Aniseed: Greeks and Romans praised aniseed for its ability to increase libido. It actually contains several compounds that are similar to estrogen, but continues to have the reputation as a male aphrodisiac.

Almond: Historically, the almond has represented fertility. Its aroma is believed to trigger sexual interest in women.

Basil: Sweet basil is believed to stimulate sexual interest and increase fertility.

Cardamom: This spice contains cineole, which is a central nervous system stimulant. Some people assume that stimulants can stimulate sexual performance also.

Chocolate: This delectable treat contains theobromine, a substance that may elevate a person's mood.

Coriander: This aphrodisiac was mentioned in the book *The Arabian Nights* as an ingredient that helps cure a childless merchant.

Fava Beans: According to herbalist James A. Duke, PhD, the fava bean was believed to have incited the Roman poet Cicero to passion. This bean contains L-dopa, which, if taken in a pharmaceutical dose, can cause priapism—a painful, persistent erection. It is difficult to eat enough beans to cause a significant reaction, though a 8–16 ounce portion may have a mild erectile effect.

Garlic: Garlic is used by many cultures to "heat" up sexual desire.

sensual shape and stimulating placebo effect. A variety of different sources, including *The Green Pharmacy*, by James A. Duke, PhD, were used to compile the food, herb, and supplement information listed below.

Ginger: Ginger, served raw, cooked, or crystallized is thought to stimulate blood flow. It is related to cardamom and may have a similar effect. It is also believed to help women increase their sexual interest.

Honey: The ancient Egyptians included honey in cures for sterility and impotence. Mead, a fermented drink made from honey, was used in medieval times to seduce fair maidens.

Licorice: Chewing on licorice root is believed to enhance sexual interest and feelings of love.

Mustard: This spice is thought to increase desire.

Olives: Green ones are rumored to increase male virility and black ones are believed to increase a woman's sex drive.

Parsley: Parsley has estrogenic properties and is believed to help increase female sexual interest.

Pine Nuts: Pine nuts have been a popular libido-enhancer since the medieval times.

Truffles: The musky scent of the truffle was believed by Greeks and Romans to stimulate sexual interest and heighten the sense of touch.

Wine: A bit of wine can relax and stimulate sexual interest, but too much can hinder sexual performance and drop blood glucose levels. If you choose to imbibe, limit your intake to 1–2 drinks only and eat some food with it to reduce its hypoglycemic effects.

Foods That May Offer a Placebo Effect Because of Their Shape

Asparagus: The phallic-looking appearance of asparagus caused many people in the ancient world to believe that it had libido-enhancing powers.

Avocado: The Aztecs believed that the shape of avocados resemble male testicles. Their name for the avocado tree was "Ahuacuatl" which means "testicle tree."

Banana: A fruit with a phallic shape.

Carrots: A vegetable with a phallic shape.

Figs: This fruit resembles female sexual organs.

Oysters: This famous aphrodisiac resembles female genitalia. In the second century, Roman satirist Juvenal, describes the sexually stimulated behavior of women who have consumed wine and "giant oysters." A word of caution: it is possible for individuals who have diabetes and other medical conditions to contract the vibrio vulnificus infection by eating raw or undercooked oysters, which are a prime transmitting agent of hepatitis. Symptoms of this infection may be vague or include:

- Gastroenteritis/abdominal pain
- Fever/chills
- Skin lesions on trunk or extremities that develop into ulcers
- Septicemia
- Hypotension
- Shock

To avoid developing this condition, do not eat any raw oysters, regardless of how they are prepared. For more information, visit *www.safeoysters.org*.

Raspberries and Strawberries: These have been highlighted in erotic literature as food items that partners feed to one another.

Aphrodisiac Recipes
Add Spice to Marriage

Jodie has had type 1 diabetes for 20 years and wants to prepare a special dinner to celebrate her 10th wedding anniversary with her husband Jack. She has an enticing diabetes-friendly meal warming in the oven, a bottle of champagne chilling in the fridge, and wants to add a bit of fun by including small amounts of foods that will enhance the evening's sexual ambiance. She searches throughout the Internet for different aphrodisiacs and decides to add oysters and an olive marinade to the menu, and she tops off her low-carbohydrate frozen dessert with a small chocolate kiss.

Can real hope be found in the world of aphrodisiacs? The answer may be found in a new synthetic drug that goes by the name Bremelanotide, which shows promise as a treatment for libido issues in both men and women. Others will certainly follow as more research becomes focused on this important topic.

SCENTS

Provocative perfume ads fill our magazines and television airwaves. Each scent claims to increase our sexual appeal to the opposite sex, but research conducted at the Smell & Taste Treatment Research Foundation in Chicago, headed by neurologist Dr. Alan Hirsch, shows that this may actually be incorrect. According to his studies published in *Medical Aspects of Human Sexuality* and other journals, floral perfume only prompted a 3% increase in blood flow to the sexual organ of men and the scent of men's cologne actually lowered blood flow to women's vaginal area. The aromas of certain foods, on the other hand, caused dramatically positive responses in both sexes.

Thirty odors were tested on 31 male subjects and their effect on penile blood flow was measured. All had an effect, but not to the same degree. As shown in the chart below, lavender and pumpkin pie prompted the greatest response. Cranberry, which stimulated the lowest response, only increased penile blood flow by 2%. They also discovered that age could

The Effects of Scents and Scent Combinations on Male Sexual Arousal

Scent	% increase in penile blood flow
Lavender and pumpkin pie	40
Doughnut & black licorice	31.5
Pumpkin pie & doughnut	20
Orange	19.5
Lavender & doughnut	18
Black licorice and cola	13
Black licorice	13
Doughnut & cola	12.5
Lily of the valley	11
Buttered popcorn	9
Cinnamon buns	4

affect preferences. For example, older men tended to respond strongly to vanilla. The chart above shows the results that were obtained in the studies run by Dr. Hirsch.

For women, the most sexually stimulating aroma was made up of a combination of Good & Plenty (a licorice-flavored candy) and cucumber. They also reacted positively to the scent of baby powder and the combination of lavender and pumpkin pie. Their sexual desire dropped, however, when they were exposed to the scents of cherries, barbeque, and men's cologne. The cherry smell may cause this negative response because of its association with the flavoring used in certain medicines and cough drops.

Dr. Hirsch believes that certain odors tap into positive memories of past experiences or are simply relaxing. Some stimulate the reticular activating system in the brain, which is responsible for arousal and motivation and causes men to become more alert to sexual cues. It is interesting to note that researchers at the Smell & Taste Treatment and Research Foundation observed that many patients who lost their sense of smell also suffered from sexual dysfunction.

The Effects of Scents and Scent Combinations on Female Sexual Arousal

Scents	% change in vaginal blood flow (turn ons)
Good & Plenty (black licorice candy) combined with cucumber	+14
Baby powder	+13
Pumpkin pie combined with lavender	+11
Baby powder combined with chocolate	+ 4
Perfume	+1

Odors	% change in vaginal blood flow (turn offs)
Cherry	-18
Charcoal-barbecued meat	-14
Men's cologne	-1

STIMULATE YOUR OTHER SENSES

What you see can stimulate the rest of your body. Men usually respond enthusiastically to a woman who is dressed seductively. Women will often respond to an attractive man. You and your partner can try to heat up your relationship by viewing a sexy video or film together. If you don't feel comfortable searching for an X-rated movie, many popular feature films contain erotic moments and can be rented without any embarrassment at all. You can also read erotic magazines or books together.

Romantic Music

Your hearing can also awaken feelings of romance. While dating, did you and your spouse have a special song? Listen to it again and feel old loving memories surface. If you don't have a favorite song, play a tune that is known for being romantic. Here are some artists who have brought romance to many couples:

- Andrea Bocelli
- Mariah Carey
- Celine Dion
- Michael Bublé
- Harry Connick, Jr.
- Josh Groban

- Faith Hill
- Tim McGraw
- Barbra Streisand
- Trisha Yearwood
- Alicia Keys
- Frank Sinatra
- Shania Twain
- Barry White

HERBAL SUPPLEMENTS

Herbal treatments for sexual complications are tempting. Many promise miracles, but can they deliver? Herbs may improve certain medical conditions for two reasons—they either contain active medicinal substances or offer a placebo effect. The main concern about herbal use is that the supplement industry is not well monitored and some products can appear safe, yet interfere with other medications or contain unsafe ingredients. If you wish to explore the use of herbs and other supplements be sure to:

- Discuss your choice of supplement with your health care team before using it. The ingredients that it contains may negatively affect medications that you currently use.
- Review the herb's safety and possible side effects at *www.medlineplus. gov*, a service of the U.S. National Library of Medicine and the National Institutes of Health.
- Look for products that are USP-verified. The United States Pharmacopeia (USP) is the official standards-setting authority for all over-the-counter and prescription medications. This approval assures you that the ingredients inside provide the value that is mentioned on the label. For a listing of USP-verified products, visit *www.usp.org*.
- Check out the safety of a particular brand of supplement at *www.consumerlab.com*. This independent testing organization reviews different products for safety and effectiveness. This is not an inclusive list of all safe supplements, but it is helpful.
- Test your blood sugar frequently. Many products can cause unexpected changes in glucose control. Treat abnormal glucose levels as directed by your health team.
- Stop using any item immediately if side effects appear.
- Discontinue all herbs and supplements several weeks prior to any surgical procedure as they may interfere with healing or other medications.

Curiosity Over Herbal Supplements

Greg stood quietly as he scanned the abundant display of herbs and supplements on the shelves of his local health food store. Lately, he has been able to achieve an erection, but it doesn't last long enough to be completely satisfying. He knows that he should say something to his doctor, but he's been friends with him for so many years, that he's uncomfortable discussing any topics other than his usual diabetes-related issues of glucose control, blood pressure, weight, and foot care. He doubts that the herbs he sees have any value, but he's still very curious about them.

The following herbs and supplements may help enhance sexual performance.

Arginine (L-arginine)

This is a popular ingredient found in supplements that claim to treat sexual dysfunction. In the body, arginine helps synthesize nitric oxide, a compound that relaxes blood vessels and permits increased blood flow to the penis. Not all studies support the use of arginine to treat men's sexual issues, but some do. Well-planned studies of the effects of arginine as a solo treatment for women have not been done, but a study at the University of Hawaii's school of medicine examined a commercial product and found that it significantly increased:

- women's sexual desire
- feeling of satisfaction with their sex life
- frequency of orgasms
- improved clitoral sensation without causing significant side effects

Ashwaganda (Withania somnifera)

This root is believed by Ayurvedic medicine experts to help improve male libido and infertility.

Butea superba

A small study performed in Thailand demonstrated the ability of this plant to help enhance erectile function in men who were approximately 70 years old. It has no known negative side effects.

Carnitine (L-carnitine)

This supplement may be able to treat male sexual issues and male infertility. One study conducted in Italy observed that two forms of carnitine improved the effectiveness of Viagra. Carnitine does not have significant side effects, but high doses may cause:

■ diarrhea
■ increased appetite
■ body odor
■ rash

Country mallow (Sida cordifolia)

This herb contains ephedrine, a stimulant that may cause men to become sexually aroused.

DHEA

Dehydroepiandosterone (DHEA) is a natural hormone that is produced by the body. Early research suggests that it may help improve sexual function and libido in women and may be helpful in men as well. These studies are just preliminary and must be expanded before any official recommendation can be made. Do not take DHEA without the guidance of a physician.

Guarana

This popular herbal drink contains a significant amount of caffeine. It is thought to be a sexual stimulant.

Yohimbe

This herb may help promote a modest increase of blood flow to the penis, but any significant improvement in sexual interest or performance is probably caused by a placebo effect. Yohimbe should not be used without a physician's approval and must be avoided by individuals with liver or kidney problems, prostate issues, or a history of gastric or duodenal ulcers. Side effects can include:

- increased anxiety
- high blood pressure
- nausea
- insomnia
- a fast heart beat
- vomiting

Ginkgo biloba

Known for its ability to improve blood flow through the brain, ginkgo biloba may also helps improve blood flow to the penis. It may take several months before any improvement is seen. Large doses can cause diarrhea.

Ginseng

Studies show that Panax ginseng enhances the synthesis of nitric oxide, which help the blood vessels in the penis relax and allow blood to enter. It also contains active ingredients called ginsenosides that encourage relaxation and may heighten a woman's sexual interest. Ginseng should be used with extreme caution if you have diabetes, as it can lower blood glucose levels and negatively affect blood pressure levels.

Maca

A 12-week Peruvian study showed that maca (lepidium meyenii), a root that is related to turnips and radishes, may help increase male sexual interest. It has no known negative side effects.

Muira puama

This Amazonian tree may help restore libido and treat erectile dysfunction. No side effects have been reported.

Oats (Avena sativa)

Stallions are fed wild oats to become friskier and libidinous, which, according to herbalist James A. Duke, PhD, is where we got the phrase "sowing wild oats." Oats may have a positive sexual effect on human males as well.

Wolfberry (Lycium Chinense)

The Chinese believe that this herb has anti-aging properties. It may raise testosterone levels in men.

SPEND TIME TOGETHER

Sometimes just being together, walking, and chatting will warm feelings of affection that can translate into heightened feelings of romance. We live extremely busy lives. We carry cell phones wherever we go and frantically run to check our email. Our hectic schedules frequently keep us from spending quality time with the one we love. Take that time to reconnect, to laugh, and enjoy life again as a pair. Set up a date night that includes a movie or walk. The more you connect outside of the bedroom, the easier it will be to connect in the bedroom.

Be open to additional ways to enhance your intimate life. Make your bedroom a place to relax and enjoy the company of a loving partner by creating an environment of fun and bonding.

FOR YOU AND YOUR PARTNER

1 How do you and your partner define intimacy? Romance?

2 What fun activities would you like to add to your intimate life?

3 What fun actions enhanced your romantic life when you first began dating each other? Would you enjoy doing them once again?

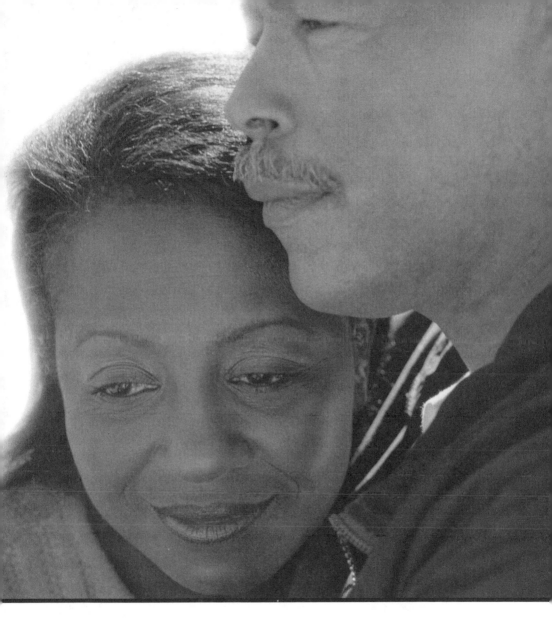

Chapter 7
For Couples

In this chapter:

▌ Evaluate how you and your partner discuss your sexual relationship.

▌ Learn how to communicate sexual concerns more effectively.

▌ Use a "magic pencil" to share your feelings.

SHARE YOUR sexual concerns with your partner. An understanding and informed loved one can offer an invaluable amount of support.

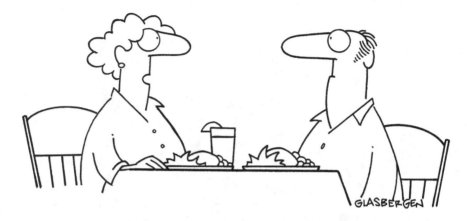

**"This is the nicest conversation we've had in weeks.
Let's not spoil it by talking."**

COMMUNICATION

How do you and your loved one discuss personal issues? See if your style of sharing fits into any of the styles of communication listed below.
- Cliff and Clair Huxtable
- Archie and Edith Bunker
- Superman and Lois Lane

Cliff and Clair Huxtable— passionate and open communication

Bill Cosby and Phylicia Rashad played Dr. Healthcliff and his wife Clair Huxtable, one of the most endearing television couples on "The Cosby Show" from September 1984 to April 1992. The Huxtables communicated on a variety of different topics with warmth and humor and openness; their bedroom pillow talk was intimate and fun. One can only assume that sexual problems would be discussed with equal clarity and affection. If you and your partner discuss sexual concerns openly, your relationship falls into this category.

Open Communication Is Key to a Successful Relationship

Scott and Jennifer enjoy a "Huxtable" relationship. They are as open about what they would like to eat for dinner as what sexual experience they would like to attempt in the bedroom. When Jennifer began feeling some dryness during intercourse, she immediately mentioned it to Scott and reassured him that her feelings toward him remained enthusiastic, so that was not cause for concern. Together, they tried to determine the cause. Jennifer visited with her doctor and began to use a vaginal lubricant. She also tested her blood sugar more aggressively to help maintain her blood sugar level in a healthier range.

Archie and Edith Bunker— lots of effort, but miscommunication

This famous, long-married couple from the television series "All in the Family" conversed a great deal, but understood very little that was shared. Personal topics frequently embarrassed them. They supported each other on many levels, but were often hampered by their own personal discomfort with intimate topics. Can you imagine Edith telling Archie that she had some pain during intercourse? Can you picture Archie speaking about potential ED concerns with Edith? If your intimate communication is not forthcoming and comfortable, your relationship falls into the Archie and Edith Bunker category.

Embarrassment Over Intimate Concerns

Betty and Connor rarely discuss intimate concerns. They have learned over their 35 years of marriage that they don't discuss sexual topics well. Connor is embarrassed by women's issues such as menstruation, childbirth, and orgasm. He calls them "women's things." When Connor had problems achieving and maintaining an erection, he told Betty that he was going to talk to his doctor about "you-know-what." When he purchased a penile pump, he was told that it could be used to enhance foreplay. He didn't invite Betty to help him use the pump. Instead he headed into the bathroom to use the pump privately before returning to the bedroom.

Superman and Lois Lane—keeping secrets

Few keep secrets from their partners better than Superman and Lois Lane. Superman (a.k.a., Clark Kent) refused to disclose his true identity and Lois Lane never shared her suspicion about Superman's real identity. Of course, the "man of steel" could never have sexually related problems, but if he did, he would definitely keep them secret. Lois Lane would never admit to having any problems either. If you keep personal concerns hidden from your partner, your relationship falls into this category.

Secrets Keeping Couple Distant

Celia and David never discuss their love life. When Celia noticed that David's desire for intimacy had dropped, she never said a word. She didn't ask if anything was bothering him or even if his diabetes had become worse. She assumed that the change was due to his increased accounting workload. If she had known that his diabetes was the cause, she could have made an effort to change their home environment to help support his diabetes needs. Instead, she just waited for tax season to end.

More effective communication

If you'd like to communicate more effectively, try the following suggestions, many of which were contributed by Yolanda Turner, EdD, Instructor of Psychology at Eastern University in St. Davids, PA, and adjunct professor in the Human Sexuality Doctoral program at Widener University, Chester, PA.

Examine your fears

If you don't feel ready to discuss a diabetes-related sexual complication with your partner, ask yourself the following questions:

1. What is stopping you from sharing this issue?
2. What do you fear will happen if you do?

After answering these questions, you may find your worries far less overwhelming. Once you feel ready to move on, follow the next steps and begin the conversation. If your concerns feel insurmountable or you are unable to pinpoint what is holding you back from having this talk, seek the help of a mental health counselor who can help you improve your perspective and move forward. Whatever you choose to do, don't pull away—that will only make matters worse.

Recognize the value of discussion

Couples who hesitate to share their feelings with each other may fear rejection, be unwilling to look honestly at their situation, or may worry that the information they disclose will harm the relationship. If done with respect and affection, your discussions should help bring you closer to your loved one. It would be lovely if your spouse could read your mind, but that rarely happens. It is easier to find solutions when you are open and honest.

Make an appointment

Set a specific time for your conversation. You won't get much accomplished and may feel hurt if your partner watches the television while you speak or is distracted by other activities.

Meet away from the bedroom

When a problem occurs during sexual activity, you may be tempted to talk about it right away, but fight the urge. Save the discussion for a later date. It could be the next day or even several weeks later. At that time, both of you will hopefully be less focused on your personal reaction to the event and will be better able to listen and offer support.

> Sexual issues can be awkward and embarrassing. Listen intently and make eye contact. Your body language will communicate how much you care.

Plan ahead

Plan your meeting by preparing a list of questions for you and your partner to discuss.

Discussion Questions

1. What is your sexual complication and why is it occurring now?
2. Whom should you see for help—your diabetes educator, urologist, physician, etc., and would your partner join you at these appointments?

Will your partner support your choice of treatment? Most options work better when a spouse adds his or her support. Pills require a waiting period and may cause a loss of spontaneity that a partner must be willing to support. Alternative sexual positions and/or the use of a vibration tool can help both men and women experience heightened sexual sensation or return some sensation that may have been lost because of diabetic neuropathy. A vacuum pump and specially prepared lubricants can be used privately in a bathroom or used with a partner to enhance sexual foreplay.

Consider your partner's feelings

After experiencing a sexual problem, you and your partner may feel a variety of different emotions.

▊ If you are a man who has just experienced an ED episode, you may feel a variety of emotions ranging from embarrassment to anger, disappointment, and frustration. No one wants to be viewed as a failure in the bedroom. Unfortunately, a failed romantic episode can lead to a fear of future failures. If you have difficulty achieving an erection, your female partner may feel rejected, disappointed, worried, guilty, or even frightened.

Many women blame themselves for their partner's inability to complete a sexual act. They worry that they may no longer be desirable or that the relationship is faltering. If she wants to become pregnant, her disappointment may be extremely intense. She may also fear that this event is the sign that more serious diabetes complications will develop.

▌ If you are a woman with diabetes who has just experienced a problem during intercourse, you may feel puzzled, upset, angry, sore, fearful, or frustrated and may not understand why this has occurred. You can't comprehend why your body suddenly won't respond or why intercourse has become so uncomfortable. Your male partner may feel rejected, disappointed, or angry. Consider your emotions and those of your partner as you prepare for your discussion.

Stay on topic

Your ultimate goal is to create an action plan. Should you try a different technique or treatment? Is it time to revisit your health care team? Is there some way for your partner to help you? Keep your comments topical. Don't bring up old business. Stay focused on your particular issue and don't bring up the past.

Don't blame yourself or each other

With diabetes, there is enough blame to go around! Some people blame themselves for ignoring health recommendations. Some blame their partner for bringing undesirable food into the home. Don't permit the conversation to turn into a blame game. If he or she begins saying how something is your fault, try to shift back to the positive. Such as how you feel when these episodes occur and how will you feel if your partner helps you? Remind your partner that your goal is to work something out for the future.

Concentrate on the good things

Find a way to weave compliments into your discussion. Hold each other's hand, if appropriate. Hug and treat each other tenderly.

Be a good listener

Don't interrupt when your partner is talking. Many couples have developed poor listening habits over the years. Think about how you feel when someone listens closely to your concerns. Sexual issues can be awkward and embarrassing. Listen intently and make eye contact. Your body language will communicate how much you care.

Use your pillow talk

Many couples have pet names for their private parts, which bond you together because they were assigned during moments of fun. Use this special language to explain your sexual problem and enlist help from your mate. These terms connect you and your partner in an intimate way that doesn't exist in any other relationship. David decided to speak to Katie about his ED. "'Willie' isn't working anymore," he said. Katie smiled and they held each other for a moment. "Let's call the doctor and see what he can do. We'll make 'Willie' feel better soon."

Be patient

This discussion may not be easy or comfortable, so be patient with each other. Communicating with a member of the opposite sex can be a challenge. Because our perspectives vary, it may take a bit of effort to get your partner to fully understand your needs and concerns.

Clashing Viewpoints

"Men and women think differently, approach problems differently, emphasize the importance of things differently, and experience the world around us through entirely different filters."—*Marianne J. Legato, MD, the author of* Why Men Never Remember and Women Never Forget

Follow up with loving gestures

After the conversation has taken place, bring flowers or a loving gift home. Invite your loved one out for a romantic picnic. Place a love note in his or her lunch or briefcase. Leave a fun message on your spouse's private voicemail. Demonstrate that the love you have for each other reaches far beyond any physical connection.

THE MAGIC PENCIL

As you discuss your concerns with your partner, you may find it helpful to use The Magic Pencil exercise recommended by Yolanda Turner. This exercise uses a pencil to determine who will share and who will rephrase. Here is how it works:

The Magic Pencil

1. Take a pencil in your hand. Say how you feel about an issue by making statements that begin with the word "I," as in "I feel," "I need," "I experience," etc.

   Shelley (holds the pencil and says): *"I feel responsible when we aren't able to finish making love. I believe that you would be able to have an erection if I were more attractive to you."*

2. Your partner then rephrases your statement using different words to express the same thought.

   Ted (rephrasing Shelley's words): *"You blame yourself when I can't perform sexually, because you think I'm not turned on by you anymore."*

3. When you are finished sharing your feelings, pass the pencil to your partner.

   It is now your partner's turn to share personal feelings in the same way that you did, using "I" statements.

   Ted (w/pencil): *"I feel that it is MY fault. I feel very attracted to you, but I feel guilty that I have diabetes."*

4. You rephrase them.

   Shelley (rephrasing Ted's words): *"You put the weight of our sexual life on yourself when your diabetes comes into our bedroom."*

(continued on page 120)

The Magic Pencil (continued from page 119)

5. Repeat this process as many times as needed. If there are any misunderstandings, clarify your thoughts.

   Ted (w/pencil): *"I feel really uncomfortable when we go out, because I have gained a lot of weight from my diabetes medications."*

   Shelley (rephrasing Ted's words): *"Your diabetes medications caused you to gain weight, so you have a harder time walking and going places."*

   Ted corrects Shelley: *"No, not exactly, it's more like I feel uncomfortable because I believe that people are staring at how heavy I am. I gained the weight from taking diabetes medications, but I feel that they think that I don't care about my health."*

   Shelley (trying again to reflect more accurately): *"OK.... What I hear you say is that you're feeling self-conscious about being heavier than you used to be, and you feel like others are judging you."*

6. You are not allowed to express any personal feelings unless you are holding the pencil. Don't judge or blame your partner for any behavior that he or she mentions. After both of you feel that you have shared adequately, begin the final round.

7. Final Round: Now it is time to take action. This round enables you to suggest a positive behavior that you can both do to improve the situation and strengthen your relationship. To do this, complete the following phrase:

   "It would be really helpful if _____."

8. Don't ask for a particular behavior to stop—that is negative. Suggest a positive and specific behavior that you both should begin. For example:

   Don't say this: *"It would be really helpful if…we could stop being too busy and distracted."*

Say this instead: *"It would be really helpful if…we could find 15 minutes a day to sit uninterrupted and talk."*

Or

"It would be really helpful if…we rode our bikes together on Saturday mornings. We could exercise and be together."

Or

"It would be really helpful if…we hired a babysitter every Saturday night so we could go out to dinner or to a movie."

Here are some other activities you can suggest in your final round or do at another time.

Attend a diabetes class

You can both learn more about diabetes together.

Watch a DVD on the topic together

The Public Health Foundation has an entertaining and educational DVD on the topic of diabetes-related complications that was prepared by dLifeTV. Watch it together. It can help launch a meaningful discussion about this important topic. It includes information about men's, women's, and couple's issues and the value of communication and caring when these problems arise. Contact the Public Health Foundation at *www.phf.org* or (202) 218-4400.

Visit a website together

Several websites offer excellent information and a bit of fun. *www.Astroglide.com* has a game and humorous story section called "Astro-fun." *www.Ky.com* offers romance stories, quizzes, and entertaining film clips, and *www.Viagra.com, www.cialis.com,* and *www.levitra.com* offer tips, quizzes, and additional information on their respective medications.

Kick start your romance with a Jump Start Pledge

In chapter 2 we introduced the use of Jump Start Pledges as a way to gently introduce new health practices into your life. This technique can also be used to infuse a bit more romance into your relationship.

How you and your loved one relate to one another is important. Try some of the suggestions listed in this chapter. If your relationship continues to be strained, meet with a qualified counselor who can help you work through this problem together.

Relationship-Building Pledges

"Between the kids and work, David and I rarely connect anymore. I've used Jump Start Pledges to help me take care of my type 1 diabetes, so I thought that I might try using them for this situation. When David comes home from work, he sits on the couch to watch old "Seinfeld" reruns as he waits for me to prepare dinner. This week, I pledged to take 15 minutes from my dinner preparations each day and cozy up to David on the couch for a part of the show. It made such a difference. That small amount of shared time has made us more affectionate. Now when he comes home from work, he searches for me and kisses me hello. This is a Jump Start Pledge that I will happily renew."—*Kristin*

FOR YOU AND YOUR PARTNER

1 How well did you and your partner communicate using the Magic Pencil exercise?

2 Share your communication strengths and weaknesses with your partner.

3 What steps can each of you take to improve your communication with one another?

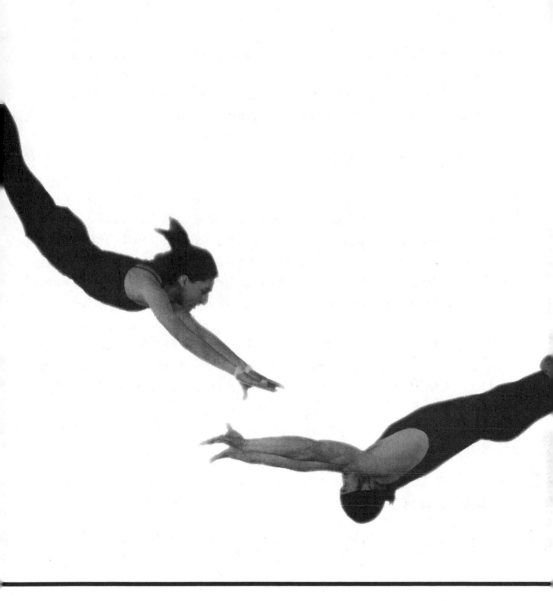

Chapter 8
Don't Try This at Home

In this chapter:

▮ Examine several bogus sexual treatments for men and women.

▮ Discover the truth about sexual products that are advertised.

▮ Learn to detect fraudulent claims.

HAVE YOU FELT tempted to purchase a treatment from a magazine, website, or sex shop? Some of the products sold are a harmless waste of money, while others may be dangerous. Let's look at some of the products that have enticed us over the years and try to tempt us today.

SEXUAL SCAMS

It is 1923 and you've just tuned your radio to the new, powerful station run by entrepreneur Dr. John Brinkley. The good doctor tells you that he has exactly what you are searching for—an effective treatment for male impotence. He implants goat glands into men's scrotums with amazing results. It sounds odd, but people say it works. Dr. Brinkley quotes research that supports him, but you want additional information. You discover that this medical wizard is no doctor at all—he purchased his medical degree, falsified his data, and has become wealthy from doing this and other procedures. As for his satisfied customers, they are being conned by the placebo effect, a belief so strong in a product's effectiveness that the user experiences an actual response.

Let's fast forward to today. Sexual scams still exist and, sadly, people continue to waste their money, harm their health, and make the charlatans who sell these items very wealthy.

Sex Scam Headlines

Here are some examples of today's advertisements for sexual stimulants. At first glance, many of the faulty ads sound enticing.

"A safe, natural, and effective sexual performance enhancer"
"Enhances libido in men and women"
"Guaranteed to work"
"Miracle cure"
"Restores the vitality of youth"

Unfortunately, they don't work. The above claims are seen on products ranging from penis enlargers, breast enhancers, and libido-heightening pills. Here is an excerpt from a recent warning that the FDA issued about several of these products.

FDA Warning Concerning Sex Scam Products

The U.S. Food and Drug Administration (FDA) is warning consumers not to purchase or consume Zimaxx, Libidus, Neophase, Nasutra, Vigor-25, Actra-Rx, or 4EVERON. These products are promoted and sold on websites as "dietary supplements" for treating erectile dysfunction (ED) and enhancing sexual performance, but they are, in fact, illegal drugs that contain potentially harmful undeclared ingredients. These products have not been approved by FDA, and there is no guarantee of their safety and effectiveness, or of the purity of their ingredients...

Consumers with diabetes, high blood pressure, high cholesterol, or heart disease often take nitrates. ED is a common problem in men with these conditions and they may seek products like the ones noted above because these products claim that they are "all natural" or that they do not contain the active ingredients used in FDA-approved ED drugs. In addition, because the manufacturing source of the active ingredients in these "dietary supplements" is unknown, there is no assurance that the ingredients are safe, effective, or pure.

Excerpt from FDA, July 17, 2006

Penis enlargement tools

Vacuum pumps

Pumps can encourage the development of an erection, but will not alter the length of the penis. Attempts to use them to enlarge the penis permanently can damage penile tissue.

Penile weights

Claim to help stretch the penis. They are not effective and can cause permanent damage.

Jelquing

Proponents of this elaborate and aggressive stretching technique claim that it permanently elongates the penis. Their claims are untrue and can cause pain and scarring.

False Products

Frank has type 2 diabetes and has been having some problems in the bedroom lately. He is a bit shy about speaking with his doctor and hoped to take care of this problem on his own. While reading a magazine, he spotted an ad for an interesting herbal penile enlargement supplement. "It's just herbs. How bad can it be?" He thought. "If it doesn't work, then I will just stop using it." The price was $39.95 for a bottle of 90 capsules, which seemed reasonable, so he sent away for one.

Here are a few of the ingredients found in the product that Frank purchased. We evaluated them by checking them out at *www.consumerlab.com*, a reliable and independent herb and supplement testing website:

Selected Ingredients Found in Frank's "100% Natural" Supplement

Horny goat weed extract: According to a report in the journal *Psychosomatics*, a 66-year-old man with a history of heart problems began to experience shortness of breath, chest pain, and irregular heart beat, after taking a daily dose of horny goat weed extract for two weeks. He reported that he had started taking a daily pill of horny goat weed to help increase his sexual experience. The experts who evaluated the case believe that the herb caused these heart-related symptoms to appear.

Saw palmetto extract: This herb can cause nausea and abdominal pain, dizziness, and headaches. Saw palmetto may also prolong bleeding and reduce platelet activity.

Tribulus terrestris extract: Studies done in Bulgaria demonstrated the safety of this herb, but the reliability of these studies have been questioned by experts. Its effectiveness is questioned as well.

Ginkgo extract: This herb may interact with other nutrients or drugs, especially if the blood-thinning drug Coumadin or aspirin is used. Some individuals may experience nervousness, headache, and stomachache.

Licorice extract: Whole licorice (herb) can cause elevated blood pressure levels if used for more than two weeks. Licorice extract may cause similar difficulty.

Nettle extract: This herb may interact with blood sugar–lowering medications.

Cayenne extract: Research done in Jamaica and published in the journal

Phytotherapy Research shows that capsaicin, one of the potent ingredients in cayenne pepper, can lower blood sugar levels. A person taking this herb preparation may experience an unexpected drop in his glucose level.

Was this product appropriate for Frank? As expected, he experienced no permanent change in penis size.

Pills

Several herbal supplement pills claim to help enlarge the penis. Herbs should not be taken cavalierly. They have medicinal properties and can interfere with other medications that you use or cause complications, such as an unexpected drop in blood sugar levels.

If you are upset about the size of your penis, you probably have nothing to worry about. According to experts at the Mayo Clinic, 70% of men have penises that measure between 5 and 7 inches when erect. A penis is considered small if it is less than 3 inches when erect. The penile enlargement tools and enlargement procedures advertised in the media today are not effective and may even damage the penis and actually cause erectile dysfunction.

Most men who seek penile enlargement have normal-sized anatomy and have no cause for concern. They should also not be concerned about how

Penis Enlargement Scams

Zack gained a lot of weight when he began using insulin to help control his type 2 diabetes. Whenever he looked in the mirror, especially after showering, he saw a sad, unattractive man with an unappealing belly hanging over his belt. His efforts to lose weight were useless. His stomach had grown so much that he was no longer able to see a particular part of his anatomy—his penis, which he found terribly upsetting. Zack decided to enlarge it and hoped that this change would make him feel better about himself. He ordered several expensive items that he spotted at the back of a magazine. All were a waste of money.

their anatomy is viewed by women. A study published in the *Archives of Sexual Behavior* found that size was not a very important concern to most of the women surveyed.

The experts at the Mayo Clinic have a suggestion that will work if you are concerned about your size—weight loss. "If your lower abdomen hangs over your genitalia, you might look as if you have a shorter, smaller penis than you actually do. Fat can obscure some or much of the upper part of the penis." Trimming the pubic hair can also help give that area a different appearance. If your weight loss efforts have been unsuccessful, seek out the help of a registered dietitian who can design a weight loss program that fits your needs.

Breast enhancers

Numerous products are being sold that claim to augment breast size—creams, sprays, and even suction tools. They can harm the fragile breast tissue and cause damage.

Vacuum

The following is an excerpt from a news release about a court action that was filed against the marketer of a "breast-enlargement" device.

Applying a vacuum to the outside of the breast might slightly stretch tissue on the surface, but it will not change the shape of cells below the skin. Stretching tissue can cause fluid build-up, similar to what happens with hormonal change during the menstrual cycle. A device might temporarily stretch the skin of the breast, but in order to achieve true enlargement, the glandular and fatty tissue inside must increase. This can only occur with cell growth in either number or size. Glands grow in response to hormones.

Growth of fibrous tissue does not enlarge the breasts. I don't see how a vacuum device would result in long-term changes to the breast that will increase its size. There may be some short-term changes in the skin, but they are unlikely to be permanent.

News release: Iowa Attorney General, Jan. 11, 2000; updated March 8, 2001.

Creams

Breast enhancement creams don't work either. In 2003, the Federal Trade Commission reached a settlement with a California-based company that marketed a dietary supplement and topical cream in different types of media—print, radio, TV, and the Internet. It promised users "Fuller, Firmer Breasts in as Little as a Few Weeks . . . Guaranteed."

Personal testimonials accompanied the ad. Interested customers were asked to call a toll-free number to order. They were offered a 90-day risk-free guarantee and were charged up to $599 for a six-month supply of this product. According to a report posted on *wwwconsumeraffairs.com*, the product did not work. The promoters were fined $22 million.

Breast Enhancement Scams

Cindy has type 1 diabetes. While growing up, she missed numerous social events and rarely dated because of her diabetes; no boys wanted to deal with her highs, lows, and frequent trips to the emergency room. Having this disease always made her feel like an unwanted outcast. Now that she is older, she believes that larger breasts will make her feel more confident about herself and get the attention that she has always wanted. To make this happen, she ordered a pricy jar of breast-enlarging cream that she read about in a fashion magazine. It irritated her skin, so she tossed it into the garbage.

Breast augmentation

Breast augmentation is not for everyone, but it can be done safely by a qualified medical professional. It is an important option for women who have had a breast removed because of injury or cancer. Some researchers believe that implants may interfere with the ability to detect cancer via mammography, but others have disputed that fact. If you wish to augment your breast size, discuss this procedure with your health care team and seek out a board-certified surgeon who has done this procedure with other women who have had diabetes. For more information, visit *www.plasticsurgery.org*—the official website of the American Society of Plastic Surgeons—and *www.breastimplantsafety.org*.

Libido enhancers

Have you ever heard of "Chinese Crocodile Penis Pills?" We hope not. According to *www.quackwatch.com*, the FDA recently cracked down on an individual who claimed to have the 2,000-year-old formula for this item, which he claimed could rejuvenate male sexual prowess. The product was a hoax.

Many fraudulent pills claim to provide the same erectile benefits as prescription products. Their ingredients can range from harmless garlic powder to dangerous doses of drugs that require supervision by a physician. One product that was recently recalled contained sildenafil citrate, the active ingredient used in Viagra. Prescriptions for Viagra should only be given to men who meet the criteria for this drug. An unsupervised, over-the-counter product that contains Viagra's active ingredient could cause a life-threatening drop in blood pressure when used by men with:

▮ diabetes
▮ hypertension
▮ heart disease
▮ other medical problems who would not qualify

Fake libido-enhancing pills exist for women as well. Many lawsuits have been filed against these companies. As with men's pills, their ingredients can affect blood sugar control and interfere with other medications.

Aphrodisiacs

In chapter 6, we suggested several aphrodisiacs that may help heighten romantic attraction. Some had real value and others offered a harmless placebo effect. There are products, however, that are not only dangerous, but have encouraged the slaughter of innocent animals.

Animal Aphrodisiac Myths

Spanish fly (cantharides) is a legendary, life-threatening aphrodisiac. It is made from dried beetle remains, which cause heightened sexual excitement as it rushes blood to the sexual organs and irritates the urogenital tract. It can also burn the mouth and throat and cause permanent damage to the kidneys and genitals, and even lead to death.

Numerous animals have been killed to retrieve parts of their bodies that are believed to have aphrodisiac properties. These claims are untrue. The following are just a few of the animal parts that were thought to have a positive sexual effect.

- rhino horn
- bear gall bladder
- raw turtle eggs
- tiger penis
- monkey brains
- shark fin
- seal and tiger genitalia

M&M Candies Myths

And now for a ridiculous aphrodisiac rumor that encouraged thievery—colored M&M's. According to *www.snopes.com*—a website that debunks Internet myths and rumors—since the creation of this chocolate treat in 1941, different significance has been attached to the different colors of this treat.

Green: aphrodisiac
Orange: good luck
Brown: bad luck
If the last one out of the bag is **yellow**: call in sick and stay home
If the last one is **red**: make a wish and it will come true

The green aphrodisiac rumor gained prominence in the 1970s. Why the green ones were singled out by consumers remains a mystery. Some believe that the color green is associated with healing and fertility. But that wasn't the rumor that caused the theft of M&M's right from the factory conveyor belt. In 1976, the FDA banned red dye #2, causing the red M&M's to be temporarily removed from the market. Being scarce prompted a new rumor—that red M&M's were the most potent aphrodisiac of all. Employees wanted to get their hands on the remaining supply, so they began pocketing them.

How to tell if an advertised remedy is a hoax

According to the FDA, the following red flags should be cause for concern.

A celebrity endorsement

Famous individuals are paid to promote products and rarely have any medical training. Don't buy an item just because your favorite television star says so. Check out all supplements and health items with your health care team.

Inadequate labeling

As an individual with diabetes, you have probably developed an eye for labels. You read them for ingredients and nutrient content. A legitimate non-prescription medication should have a label that explains its purpose, how to use it, and when to seek medical help. Avoid products that are missing this information.

A secret formula

Walk away from a product that claims to work because of its secret formula.

Suspicious ad placement

If a product is only promoted in the back pages of magazines, by direct mail, over the phone, in newspaper ads, in mock magazine stories, or in 30-minute infomercials that masquerade as talk show interviews, it is probably a fraudulent item.

It makes impossible claims

Stay away from cure-all products that claim to improve numerous physical ailments, provide a cure that is being kept from the public by the medical establishment, have no side effects, work instantly (and permanently!), and eliminate the need for medical treatment.

THE ROLE OF THE FDA

If these products are so dangerous, why are they still on the market?

In 1994, President Clinton signed the Dietary Supplement Health and Education Act (DSHEA), which made manufacturers and distributors responsible for safety of their dietary supplements and the accuracy of the claims that they made. They did not need FDA approval before placing an item on the market unless a new dietary ingredient was introduced. It is up to you to take the extra time to review any supplement or product that you wish to use with your health care team before you try it.

The FDA and the U.S. Federal Trade Commission (FTC) work tirelessly to stop the sale of phony products, but it is a gargantuan task. The Internet is an unmonitored, international marketplace where new items are posted every day. Help remove hazardous products from the marketplace.

Reporting Phony Products to the FDA and FTC

▮ Report negative medical effects at: *www.fda.gov/medwatch*.
▮ Report problems that don't involve a serious or life-threatening reaction at: *www.fda.gov/oc/buyonline/buyonlineform.htm*.
▮ To report emails or websites that promote illegal medical products, forward the material to: *webcomplaints@ora.fda.gov*.
▮ To report false claims to the Federal Trade Commission, call (877) 382-4357.

Don't waste your hard-earned funds on products that make big promises, but deliver dangerous or inadequate results. It is tempting to search for an easy fix, but they rarely exist. Your health and intimate relationship are worth quality attention. Make the effort to get the help that you deserve.

FOR YOU AND YOUR PARTNER

1 List any questionable sexual remedies you or your partner have tried. Have you shared this information with your partner?

2 Why is it important to review the safety of your remedy choices with a qualified health care professional?

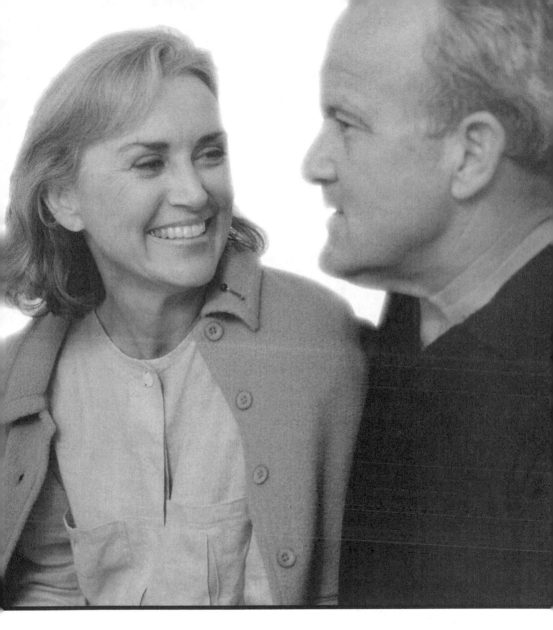

Chapter 9
As We Age

In this chapter:

▮ Identify the natural changes that happen to our bodies as we age.

▮ Learn about the changes that may develop because of diabetes.

▮ Review ways to keep your mind and body ready for love.

▮ Explore a different approach to intimacy.

INTIMATE RELATIONSHIPS are not only for the young. As we age, we can still enjoy a passionate life, even with diabetes. Our need to be connected physically with another human being doesn't diminish when the hair on top of our head develops a touch of grey or we begin to wear reading glasses. But our lovemaking, as well as the quality of many of our physical activities, will be different. Whether we have diabetes or not, our bodies are destined to change as we become older and alter how we perform sexually.

Sexual Functions As We Age

20–30 years	trice daily
30–40 years	tri weekly
40–50 years	try weekly
50–60 years	try weakly
60–70 years	try oysters
70–80 years	try anything
80–90 years	try to remember

A touch of humor from *AADE—New Perspectives on Erectile Dysfunction*, 1999

NORMAL EFFECTS OF AGING

Cartoon characters have the luxury of staying young forever. If they did age, Wilma and Fred Flintstone and Betty and Barney Rubble would appear dramatically different. Let's imagine how these two loving couples might appear if they began to age.

If Cartoon Characters Aged

Fred is now even heavier as his metabolism has slowed significantly. He has high blood pressure because his blood vessels are now less elastic and narrowed from an accumulation of fatty deposits. He also has some constipation problems, because his body now produces a smaller amount of digestive juices. Poor Barney's prostate is enlarged, so he needs to run to the bathroom often.

Betty has become a bit forgetful and sometimes loses her balance. The number of neurons in our brain decreases as we age, which affects our coordination and our memory. We adapt to some of these changes by increasing the amount of connections that exist between brain cells, but that only occurs in limited areas. Wilma wears reading glasses and her eyes feel dry, because she produces fewer tears. She is now a few inches shorter; her bones have started to shrink in size and density. Both couples raise their voices when they speak to one another, because their hearing isn't what it used to be.

All four of them have lost some muscular flexibility. They produce less saliva to rinse away cavity-producing bacteria and must visit their dentist more frequently. Both couples have also developed the outward signs of aging—wrinkles, age spots, skin tags, and gray hair, but one thing that hasn't changed is their desire for romance, closeness, and intimacy.

The following are some additional changes that can happen as women enter their menopausal years and men grow older.

Symptoms of Aging

Symptoms of perimenopause and menopause (in women)

❙ Menstrual changes

❙ Vaginal dryness

❙ Sleep problems and unusual dreams

❙ Hot flashes and/or flushes; night sweats

❙ Mood swings

❙ Fluctuations in sexual desire and sexual response

❙ Weight changes

❙ Chills or periods of extreme warmth

❙ Bouts of rapid heartbeat

❙ Frequent urination and urinary leaking during coughing, sneezing, or orgasm

(continued on page 138)

Symptoms of Aging (continued from page 137)

- Tingling in hands
- Vaginal infections
- Depression
- Painful intercourse
- Migraine headaches

Symptoms of male aging

- A drop in testosterone level
- Reduced bone strength
- Decreased muscle strength
- Decreased penile sensitivity
- A drop in libido
- A reduction in memory and concentration
- Less firm erections
- Longer time between erections
- Shorter orgasm duration
- Less forceful ejaculations
- Frequent urination (prostate problems)
- Reduced sperm production
- Hair loss
- Weight gain

If some of the symptoms sound oddly familiar, it may be because several can also be caused by diabetes. For example, frequent urination may be a symptom of an elevated blood sugar level. A feeling of extreme warmth (burning) or tingling may appear when diabetes neuropathy develops. Nightmares can occur if your blood sugar drops low during the night, and weight gain, vaginal dryness, depression, headaches, decreased libido, mood swings, and erection problems can also be related to less than optimal diabetes control.

If you develop physical or emotional changes that interfere with your ability to enjoy intimacy, ask yourself a very important question: is the problem because you've grown older or because of your diabetes? To be on the safe side, always check your physical health before you causally dismiss a problem as an inevitable sign that you are getting older. Here are several changes that may develop along with suggested ways to handle them.

You may develop bad breath

Breath Discomfort

Frank has very unappealing breath odor. He takes breath mints, but they don't do much good. Because of this, he now stays several feet away from others when he speaks. Intimacy is out of the question—he is sure that no one wants to be near him. His breath has become a real problem.

In chapter 3, we learned that individuals with diabetes can develop unpleasant ketone-scented breath when fat is used as energy by the body. There are other causes as well. Many older individuals take a generous assortment of medications that can interact with each other and cause bad breath. Dental problems, such as gum infections, may also cause this problem. Here is how you can approach this issue:

▌ Review your medications with your health care team.

▌ Visit your dentist for a cleaning/exam at least every six months.

▌ Brush regularly, floss daily, and clean your tongue gently with a tongue cleaner.

▌ If you use a mouthwash, choose one that does not contain alcohol, which can be drying to your gums. If you wish, you can create your own low-cost mouthwash—just dilute a portion of hydrogen peroxide with half of that amount of water. For example, 1 cup of hydrogen peroxide mixed with ½ cup of water.

Your sleep needs may change

It is common for older individuals to head to bed at an earlier hour and sleep less soundly. By the age of 75, some adults report that they are waking up several times each night. This could be caused by a natural change in sleep schedule, urinary incontinence, or symptoms of an elevated blood sugar level that occurs if your diabetes changes.

Interrupted Sleep

After going to bed at a very early hour, Lydia wakes up and tiptoes to the bathroom and back to bed. She does this several times throughout the night. She seems to get enough rest, but doesn't enjoy the fact that she no longer sleeps through the night. Her blood sugar has become more difficult to control, but she doesn't believe that her diabetes has caused this change to occur—her control was never a problem before.

Diabetes is often called a "progressive disease," which means that the approach you always used to control your diabetes may suddenly stop working. For example, if you always controlled your type 2 diabetes with oral medication, you may now need to use insulin to maintain the same healthy blood sugar level. This doesn't mean that you've been lax about your care or have done something wrong. As you age, your body changes and so does your diabetes—your approach to care needs to be adjusted as well. Improved blood sugar control may not keep you from waking through the night, but it should stop your need to urinate frequently if diabetes is the cause.

Your hearing may change

One out of every three individuals over the age of 60 experience some level of hearing loss. After the age of 85, half of us will have hearing loss. Hearing loss can make communication between two individuals more challenging. During intimate moments, most individuals use a soft voice or a whisper to communicate personal needs and wants. You may have to speak louder or more clearly to have a meaningful conversation.

You may develop urinary incontinence

Thirteen million male and female Americans of all ages, with and without diabetes, deal with the problem of urinary incontinence. According to experts at the Mayo Clinic, 30% of people age 65 or older will have a decrease in bladder control. There are four types of urinary incontinence—stress, urge, mixed, and overflow—that can develop.

Disrupted Sleep from Urinary Problems

Sam frequently feels the urge to run to the bathroom, but isn't able to urinate very much once he's there. He has type 1 diabetes and hasn't always been the best patient. "I was in denial for a long time. My doctor, friends, and family used to yell at me about it. I always knew that I would probably start having some sort of complication when I got older, but didn't know that I could have this type of bathroom problem. I'm really tired of this."

Four Types of Urinary Incontinence

Stress: Urine leaks when you cough, laugh, sneeze, or move in any way that puts stress on the bladder. This type occurs when the pelvic muscles and tissues become stretched or damaged from pregnancy, aging, weight gain, or certain sports—such as running and gymnastics—in which the body hits the ground with a lot of force.

Urge: This is also known as an overactive bladder. Your body sends you very little notice when you need to go. Your urge could range from just a few seconds to a minute before you experience an involuntary loss of urine. A urinary tract infection can cause this to develop.

Mixed: This is a combination of stress and urge incontinence. Most women, especially those who have had a hysterectomy, tend to develop this form. Women who have entered menopause and begin hormone replacement therapy may initially experience a temporary leaking problem that should cease as the body adjusts to a new hormone level.

Overflow: If you visit the bathroom often, but only experience a slight flow of urine whenever you go, you are experiencing overflow. Diabetic neuropathy can cause this type to develop. Men who have prostate problems may also experience this.

An effective way to improve genital muscle tone and decrease urinary leaking is to do an exercise known as "the kegel" (kay'-gul).

These exercises were initially designed by Dr. Arnold Kegel as a way to help women tone their vaginal muscles and achieve orgasm easier. They can also help avoid urinary leaking during the day and during sexual activity and help men strengthen the area around the penis, improve the quality of an erection, and help delay ejaculation just before orgasm.

Kegel Exercises

To do the kegel, first locate your pubococcygeus (PC) muscle. Head to the bathroom and begin to urinate. Stop the flow of urine several times. Each time you do, you are contracting your PC muscle. Don't squeeze your abdominal muscles, only your PC muscle. Once you identify the sensation, you can strengthen this muscle by squeezing it throughout the day. Here are several routines that you can try:

1. Squeeze your PC muscle for three seconds and release for three seconds. Repeat six times. Do this series three times each day. Gradually increase the amount of times that you do this until you repeat the exercise 12 times a day.
2. Squeeze your PC muscle strongly for a single second and release for one second. Repeat 20 times. Do this version three times each day.
3. Squeeze the PC muscle for 10 seconds. Focus on the intensity of the contraction. Repeat this five times. Do this version three times each day.

The kegel can be done anytime, anywhere. You should notice a difference after one month.

You may experience menopause-related vaginal pain

As a woman ages, her ability to achieve orgasm doesn't change, but other physical changes will take place. She may take between one to three minutes longer to lubricate following sexual stimulation than the 10–30 second rapid release of lubricant that occurred when she was younger. The mucus that is released will be thinner and less protective during intercourse. This can cause a woman to experience a significant amount of discomfort.

Exploring Options

"The creams weren't working for me. I tried them all. The pain that I experienced during intercourse was deep inside in an area that creams and lotions couldn't reach. My doctor suggested that I use a small lubricant suppository. It worked." —*Daisy*

To deal with this, enjoy a longer period of foreplay to help stimulate your body's own natural lubrication. If you feel discomfort, try one of the vaginal lubricants discussed in chapter 5. If the pain is located deep inside, your doctor may recommend an aspirin-sized, hormone-releasing lubricant pill (Vagifem) with an applicator or Estring, a ring that is placed high up in the vagina that releases estrogen over a period of about three months. After that time, it is removed and discarded. Both Vagifem and Estring are easy to use.

You may be shy about sexual activity following a heart attack

Nervous About Heart Risks

Kent's diabetes affected his heart and circulation. He knew that he should lose weight and follow a diet, but he didn't do it. After he had a small heart attack, he began to take all of the health advice that he received very seriously. He wanted to continue to enjoy intimacy with his wife, but wasn't sure if this was alright or not. His wife was very nervous about it.

People with diabetes are two to four times more likely to develop cardiovascular disease, which can lead to a heart attack or stroke. Hopefully, this will not happen, but if it does, according to the American Heart Association, you can continue to enjoy an intimate relationship with your partner. Speak with your physician and cardiac rehab team about ways to safely reintroduce sexual activity into your relationship. If you experience chest pain during or after sexual activity, you may need to take nitroglycerin or a related medicine. While taking nitroglycerin or any other nitrate-containing medicine, oral ED medications, such as Viagra, are not recommended. Fortunately, there are many other effective options to choose from. Chapter 4 discusses many of them.

You may be alone

Many individuals enter their later years without a partner. Their spouse may be deceased, the couple may be divorced, or he or she may not have married. Their re-entry into the world of sexual intimacy after a long period of celibacy, often called "Widower's Syndrome," is not always easy. A new relationship can be very stressful and cause a man to have erection problems.

Many experience performance anxiety when they return to the sexual arena. If you focus exclusively on your sexual technique, however, you may miss out on the rich connection that can develop with a new partner. If you are a woman, your vaginal muscles may need time to stretch in order to comfortably accommodate this sexual activity again. Try a variety of intimate positions, use a lubricant, and be patient.

AIDS in the Elderly

According to the National Institute on Aging: "Older people are at increasing risk for HIV/AIDS and other STDs. About 10% of all people diagnosed with AIDS in the United States—some 75,000 Americans—are age 50 and older. Because older people don't get tested for HIV/AIDS on a regular basis, there may be even more cases than we know. In addition, older people are less likely than younger people to talk about their sex lives or drug use with their doctors, and doctors don't tend to ask their older patients about sex or drug use. Finally, older people often mistake the symptoms of HIV/AIDS for the aches and pains of normal aging, so they are less likely to get tested. Women who no longer worry about getting pregnant may be less likely to use a condom and to practice safe sex. Also, vaginal dryness and thinning often occurs as women age. When that happens, sexual activity can lead to small cuts and tears that raise the risk for HIV/AIDS."

If you don't wish to jump onto the dating bandwagon, you can still participate in personal sexual gratification. Sexual activity of any type helps:

▮ release stress

▮ brings a feeling of well-being

▮ keeps the genital area of the body functioning well

If you start dating again, you may need to share your medical information. Diabetes is quite common in older individuals, so it shouldn't alter your dating options when you disclose that you have it. Always use a condom to protect yourself from sexually transmitted diseases.

You may dislike your physical appearance

Aging is rarely kind. Wrinkles appear, hair turns gray, necks sag, and bodies develop lumps and bumps in areas that used to be toned and taut. If you look in the mirror and are saddened by the loss of youth, find an activity that can help you develop new confidence in your appearance and attractiveness. One such activity is belly dancing, which encourages participants to feel agile and lovely.

Dancing for All Ages

"I admit it. I'm hooked on belly dancing. What grabbed me wasn't the lively music that ranges from Middle Eastern to rock, or the movements that tone muscles I never knew I had. I was moved by the unconditional acceptance of every individual who participates. Beginning dancers at my South Beach studio range from teens to early 70s and their figures run from healthy to quite overweight. You don't have to look perfect as you begin your quest for a healthier body here. You actually need a bit of jiggle, to look better when you wiggle! But as you progress, you will meet your personal goals. All in all, belly dancing is pure fun, a great way to burn calories, and a darned good workout."

—Excerpt from an article posted on *www.dearjanis.com*

If you are a man who wants to take your appearance to the next level, try weight training. It not only helps redefine your muscles, it can strengthen and tone your upper body, which supports you in different sexual positions. Weightlifting injuries are common, so learn how to do the repetitions properly from a trained professional at a health club or on an exercise DVD. All physical activity:

■ releases uplifting endorphins
■ improves your muscle tone
■ reduces stress
■ improves flexibility
■ can make you feel younger and more energetic
■ can help improve your diabetes control
■ improves overall health

"Are there drawbacks to getting older? Of course there are. But let me say categorically, when it comes to the subject that is my area of expertise, S E X, there's a lot of good news. Many people discover they have some of the best sex of their lives after 50, 60, and even after 70."
—Dr. Ruth, from *Dr. Ruth's Sex After 50—Revving up the Romance, Passion, and Excitement*

INTIMACY

Intimacy is more than intercourse. Touching and cuddling can turn a cold winter's night into an evening to remember.

Intimacy In Later Years

Daphne and Roger have been married for 47 years. Daphne has type 1 diabetes. She is slender, has long gray hair, and has a face that is lined with evidence of a life well lived. To Roger, she is as lovely as the day they married. "I still want us to be together. She is my love. I don't care how time has changed her body. I only see her inner strength and beauty. Our sex life isn't about athletic prowess or performance. It is about holding, caressing, and connecting. I wouldn't trade it for the world."

As we age, men and women seem to begin to share a similar appreciation for intimate activity. Many older men discover that they don't need to have an erection to enjoy orgasm. According to Georgia Witkin, PhD, the author of *Sex: the Simple Truth—Why It's Better Now*, only 17% of women in their 70s or 80s feel that intercourse is necessary for "good sex." Here are some additional facts from Dr. Witkin.

- According to a survey of 800 elderly couples, 75% of those who are still sexually active say that their lovemaking has improved.
- Almost 50% of men in their 80s say they are still interested in sex.
- Although, at 80, just one woman in five will have a sex partner, women at 80 still have the capacity for orgasm.

AADE-7 SELF CARE

To age well, it is important to maintain good health and diabetes control. In chapter 2, we introduced the Jump Start Pledge as a way to achieve personal health goals. Here is another way—the AADE-7.

Behavior change can be overwhelming, especially if you have a number of goals that you wish to achieve. The AADE-7 self-care behavior list was created by The American Association of Diabetes Educators as a way for individuals of all ages who have diabetes to set health goals and review their personal progress. A diabetes educator can help you use this list to make realistic and meaningful lifestyle changes. They include:

1. Healthy eating
2. Being active
3. Monitoring
4. Taking medications
5. Problem solving
6. Healthy coping
7. Reducing risks

Here are some ways to use each of these behaviors to keep your body healthy as you grow older.

Healthy eating

Confusion Over Weight Loss

"I've gained a lot of weight over the past year and now have a lot of trouble being with my wife—I'm too heavy and make her uncomfortable when we are in bed together. Because I have type 2, I'm not supposed to skip any meals. How will I lose the weight if I have to eat all the time?"—*Craig*

Your ability to participate in pleasurable activities, including sexual intimacy, will improve if you are well nourished and at a healthy weight. You will feel energized and have an easier time relating intimately to the one you love. A properly designed meal plan can also help you meet your personal weight goals. Tips for eating healthy are:

▌ make wise food choices
▌ reduce your portion sizes (if necessary)
▌ follow a meal plan that fits your lifestyle and medical goals.

It is a challenge to find the right balance. Fortunately, there are many ways to design a diabetes meal plan. Some are more restrictive and others are more flexible; one size does not fit all. If you are on a program that is too difficult to follow, you may crave foods that you prefer not to eat, so meet with a registered dietitian who can help design a plan that will work with your lifestyle.

Being Active

Sticking with Exercise

"I try to do some exercise every day. I usually walk outside, but when the weather is bad, I head out to an indoor shopping mall. There are lots of walkers there. I even started to recognize a few—we wave hi as we pass each other. I started wearing a pedometer that counts my steps. It makes my walking more enjoyable. I compete with myself and try to beat my goal every day."—*Fran*

Walking, swimming, and dancing are all excellent activities. Sexual activity is also a form of exercise that connects you more intimately to your partner, burns unwanted calories, stimulates healthy blood circulation, engages different muscles, and releases endorphins that lift your spirit. All forms of exercise can help lower your blood sugar level for up to 48 hours and may help you reduce your need for diabetes medication.

Monitoring

Accepting Help with Diabetes

"I used to hate my glucose monitor. I mean really hate it. It yelled at me, so I would yell back at it! But then I realized that it was helping me. It warned me if I started to go off track. If it said that my blood sugar level was high, I would take a correction dose of insulin, go for a gentle walk, and drink some water. If I was low, I would eat 15 grams of carbohydrates, wait 15 minutes, then test again. This all keeps my blood sugar level where it needs to be and that helps me keep complications from developing. Now that's pretty helpful, if you ask me. My glucose monitor is the best friend that I have."—*Van*

Information helps you make quality diabetes care decisions. Learn how to check your blood glucose on a regular basis and use the results to make more effective health care decisions. Meet with your health care provider to discuss ways to incorporate this practice into your health care plan.

Taking Medications

If you are not content with your level of control, review your medication options with your health care provider. Most people can improve their control, regardless of their age or how long they have had diabetes. New types of insulin are available as well as other injected medications such as Byetta and Symlin.

PROBLEM SOLVING

Getting to the Root of the Problem

"My morning blood sugar level made me furious each day. Whatever I did, it would go high. I tried eating a green apple before bed, but that didn't work. I took a few spoonfuls of apple cider vinegar at night, but that didn't help. Heck, I tried everything that I read on every diabetes chat room and bulletin board. Finally, I asked my doctor for help. He told me that my blood sugar level was climbing as a reaction to a group of hormones that my body releases while I sleep at night—it wasn't my fault at all. She told me that there was a great medicine that I could try. I started taking Metformin and really noticed a huge improvement. Now I start off my day feeling much more positive."—*Linda*

If you have any questions about living with diabetes, seek help. Members of your health care team are there to help guide you, but they can't do it without honest and open input from you. Chapter 10 contains suggestions that can help you communicate personal issues to your health care provider.

Ask Questions

"I had trouble controlling my blood sugar during and after sexual activity, but I never mentioned it because it was too embarrassing. My wife finally urged me to speak up. When I did, my diabetes educator told me that I shouldn't start romantic activity until my blood sugar level is at least 140. That made such a difference."—*Sid*

Healthy Coping

Having diabetes is not easy. If you find that you are feeling depressed, angry, or guilty, examine the way that you currently care for your disease, a qualified mental health professional can help you cope. Don't delay. Your emotional health can affect every part of your life, including how you relate to your partner.

Physical and Emotional Dilemmas

"Diabetes is breaking up my marriage. I haven't been feeling great, so I've taken a lot of time off from work. Now my wife is furious at me. She can't understand why I sometimes have to stay home. She is threatening to leave me if I can't get my life straightened out. We had some problems before I was diagnosed, but now things are so much worse." —*Carl*

Reducing Risks

You can reduce your risk for all types of diabetes-related complications, including sexual ones, by taking a proactive approach toward your diabetes. Set personal goals with the help of your health care team. Visit with them on a regular basis and report problems that you are having and discuss possible solutions. Unlike most medical problems, diabetes responds positively to even the smallest amount of effort. Small steps can make a huge difference.

Diabetic complications, such as neuropathy, can impair a person's ability to feel sensations that he or she enjoyed in the past. As you have already learned, there are many different treatment options for all individuals with diabetes-related sexual complications. These can be used by most individuals at any age. If you aren't currently satisfied with your intimate relationship, seek help from a qualified health professional.

"When we are young, sex is often a regular part of daily life. It is frequently in our thoughts and is a way to experience pleasure, release tension, and express feelings for a partner. For many of us, it is more physical than anything else. But as we mature, and as we build long-term relationships, sex becomes more than just a physical exercise. It can take on added levels of meaning and emotion and as a result, can have a far deeper and more significant role in our lives."—*Sex Over Forty*. October, 1992.

FOR YOU AND YOUR PARTNER

1 Review the AADE-7 list of self-care behaviors.

2 In which areas are you doing well?

3 Which areas would you like to discuss with members of your health care team? Remember, the healthier you are, the better your sex life will be.

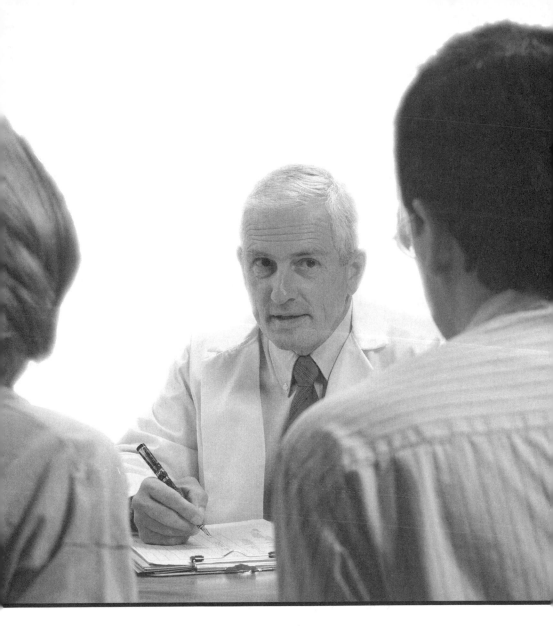

Chapter 10
Speaking with Your Doctor

In this chapter:

▌ Discover why most people don't seek help for sexual problems.

▌ Learn why health care providers may not ask about them.

▌ Find ways to help cross this communication divide.

REASONS WHY
WE DON'T ASK FOR HELP

Few individuals speak to their health care providers about sexual concerns. To make matters even more challenging, few health care team members inquire about them. Because of the difficulty of this situation, there are scenarios provided throughout this chapter with tips on how to communicate with your doctor about sexual concerns.

Medical environment

There are several reasons why many of us, patient and health care provider alike, find it difficult to speak about sexual concerns. The first is our medical environment. Over the past several years, the medical world in the United States has become rushed and impersonal. We wait for hours in boring waiting areas only to see care providers who have little time to spend with us. In an ideal world, we would all be patients of the famous 1960s television doctor Marcus Welby. Dr. Welby and his protégé, Dr. Kiley, spent generous amounts of time learning about their patients' workload, family, and other personal concerns. They never rushed anyone through a visit and quickly picked up on hints that suggested an embarrassing problem. Unfortunately, few "Dr. Welbys" exist today.

Talking to Your Doctor: Scenario 1

Dave decided to bring up the topic of ED at the start of his appointment, so that there would be plenty of time to discuss it. He said the following when his doctor entered the exam room—"Hi Doc, when you have a chance, I need to discuss a personal problem that I've been having." His physician picked up the hint immediately and addressed his concerns during the visit.

Even if you meet with a professional who provides personal care, it is still extremely difficult to fit in all of the routine topics that should be covered at each visit:

- your physical condition
- lab results

∎ weight changes
∎ medication effectiveness

This leaves little time to discuss sexual health. Providers should ask about it, but very few do. If you want to get help with your sexual complication, you should take the initiative and speak up.

Talking to Your Doctor: Scenario 2

Rhonda wants her physician to ask about her change in libido; she is too shy to bring it up herself. To make that happen, she wrote a brief letter describing her need to talk and dropped it off at the physician's office. The note said the following:

Dear Doctor Rogers,
  I'm having some problems of a sexual nature. My interest has dropped dramatically. I would like to know if it is caused by my diabetes. Can we discuss this at my next visit? I am scheduled to see you next Tuesday.
                                                                    —Rhonda D.

Her doctor received the letter and reviewed the topic during Tuesday's visit.

Embarrassment

A second impediment to discussing this topic that both patients and health care providers share is embarrassment. We talk openly about rashes and sore throats, but often feel very uncomfortable when it comes to talking about sex. At a recent conference in Miami, a group of health care providers were asked to raise their hands if they routinely inquire about the sexual health of their patients. Only a few hands went up. The rest of the audience glanced awkwardly at the floor.

So if your health care provider isn't going to mention the topic, you need to. But don't wait until the end of your visit. Some call sexual complications "doorknob issues"—topics that patients don't have the courage to bring up until their doctor has his or her hand on the doorknob and is about to leave the room. The problem with waiting until the end of the visit to say anything is that the issue may not receive the attention it deserves.

Embarrassing Situation

Lana sat nervously waiting for the doctor. She read in a magazine about how diabetes had affected one woman's sex life and wondered if her type 2 diabetes could be causing her pain during intercourse. She wanted to mention this to her doctor, but stayed silent. Sex was something that was never discussed in her family and she didn't know how to open the conversation. As her appointment came to an end, her physician started to leave the room. She finally said, "Doctor Smith, I need to talk to you about something." He looked at his watch and asked if she could wait in his office while he checked on another patient. Lana told him that it wasn't that important and went home.

Misconceptions about disease

A third reason why some people with diabetes remain silent is because they assume that their diabetes complications are inevitable—they accept their fate and don't even ask for help. Over the years, they may have ignored their diabetes, received poor care, or have had such a challenging case of diabetes that numerous complications have developed.

Giving Up Hope

Sam doesn't care anymore. He hasn't cared for a long time. He felt restricted by diabetes diets, so he didn't follow any meal plan. He never enjoyed exercising, so that recommendation was ignored. Sam also chose not to monitor his blood sugar. He has type 2 diabetes and never took it seriously. He soon developed high blood pressure and had to have two toes amputated. When he started to have problems achieving an erection, he added it to the list of important things that diabetes was stealing from him. He doesn't believe that any treatment will work for him, so he doesn't plan to mention this problem to his doctor.

If you believe that you have no hope, revisit your health care team. Diabetes treatment options have improved dramatically over the past few years and can help you improve many of the diabetes issues that you already have, and help avoid additional ones in the future. Don't let diabetes steal the physical connection that you have with a loved one.

What if you have tried to talk to your health care provider already, but have found him or her unhelpful?

Letting Embarrassment Rule Your Life

Tony has type 2 diabetes and was having frequent problems achieving an erection. At a recent visit to his doctor, he mumbled something about having a personal problem and received an equally cryptic response. His doctor nodded his head and winked, picked up his prescription pad, and silently wrote out a prescription for Viagra. No meaningful discussion took place. No directions were offered and no plan for follow-up was mentioned. At future appointments, the doctor never asked if the Viagra had worked. Unfortunately it hadn't, and because of the initial awkwardness of that first visit, Tony chose not to bring it up again. He just accepted the fact that his sex life was over.

Don't give up hope of solving your problems. The following are suggestions you can try when talking to your doctor.

When you call for an appointment, say that you may need extra time

The office manager knows the ebb and flow of the office and should be able to schedule your exam during a slower time of day. If your next appointment isn't for several months, don't wait. Schedule one to discuss your sexual concerns. You would come in if you had a mysterious, lingering cough, stubborn fever, or bruised rib. Set a time to speak about this topic.

Do some research before seeing the doctor

Read through different books and reliable websites. Note treatments that appeal to you and your partner. Ask specific questions based on your research. Instead of asking, "How can you help me?" pose a question such as, "Do you think we would benefit from seeing a sex therapist?" or "Which of my medications may be affecting my erections?"

Talking to Your Doctor: Scenario 3

Kevin has tried to discuss his ED with his doctor many times, but something always gets in the way—the phone rings, the doctor's beeper goes off, a nurse walks in, etc. So he decided to take an alternate approach and bring his concerns to another member of his health care team. His diabetes educator always asks about the stresses in his life, so he asked her to suggest a treatment for his ED. She discussed several options. Some required a prescription, but others such as vacuum pump and constriction ring, could be purchased without one. Kevin decided to buy a pump. If it doesn't work for him, he'll try something else.

Assume that your health care providers won't bring up the topic

We've already mentioned several reasons why health care professionals may not ask about your sexual issues. It will probably be necessary for you to open up the topic. If your primary care physician can't provide answers that satisfy you, don't become frustrated; there are other options for both men and women. Women can ask their primary care provider, an OBGYN, and an endocrinologist. Men can ask a primary care provider, endocrinologist, and their urologist. Your endocrinologist may know much more about the topic than you'd think. Endocrinologists specialize in male and female hormonal issues, which often have a great impact on sexual function. And, of course, they also specialize in any problems that arise from diabetes.

There are also clinicians who specialize in sexual function, such as sex therapists. Check out the resource section in the back of this book for ways to locate these different specialists.

Talking to your doctor: Scenario 4

Like Rhonda in scenario #2, Fred didn't want to be the one to bring up the topic of sex. Instead, he asked the office nurse to send the message: "Diane, please let Dr. Johnson know that I think I need a prescription for Viagra or whatever he thinks will work for me." Diane placed the message in his medical chart and also made a personal comment to the doctor. His doctor brought up the topic during Fred's appointment.

Don't be afraid

You aren't the first person to ask about sexual issues and certainly won't be the last!

Write down your questions and concerns ahead of time

This will help you remember the most valuable points to share during the visit. If you are a man, tell the doctor if you have any of these issues:

▌ erectile dysfunction
▌ poor sexual desire (decreased libido)
▌ ejaculation problems
▌ relationship problems

If you are a woman, let the doctor know if you have any of the following:

▌ poor sexual desire (decreased libido)
▌ trouble with orgasms
▌ difficulty with genital stimulation
▌ difficulty with mental stimulation
▌ pain with intercourse
▌ vaginal dryness

Mention your need to talk at the start of the session

Tell your care provider that you have something personal to discuss. He or she should get the hint.

Present your personal story in a concise and organized way

Get right to the point. It will save time during the visit and improve the chances that you'll get the treatment you need.

Ways to help cross the communication divide

The following describes a visit between George and his physician, "Dr. Neverlisten." See how many communication problems you can identify that could make it more difficult for George to successfully discuss his sexual concerns. Then try to come up with ways to deal with them.

Communication Divide

George and his wife Connie arrive at Dr. Neverlisten's office for a regular visit. He has an ED problem, but doesn't want anyone to know about it. He is a proud man and his ED makes him feel like a failure. Connie hopes that her presence will help George find the courage to talk about the problem. George hopes that his doctor will ask about it, so he doesn't have to be the one to bring it up. A nurse enters the exam room to take his vitals—blood pressure, temperature, and weight, etc. George smiles and says a quick hello. Dr. Neverlisten arrives, but immediately leaves to take a phone call. He re-enters the room, gives George a quick physical exam. "How are you doing, George?" George asks the doctor to check his right foot; he has been having some numbness lately. The doctor takes a quick look then pops back into the hallway to ask a nurse to attend to a problem. Dr. Neverlisten stops in the room to hand George a new prescription. The nurse pops her head into the room and tells Dr. Neverlisten that he has a phone call, so he leaves. From the hallway, he calls out, "Take care, George. See you in three months. Regards to the family." And he's gone. The topic of ED never comes up.

How many communication problems did you locate in the story above? Here are a few that we identified.

1. **George doesn't want anyone to learn about his ED.**
   Possible solution: If George doesn't say anything, he can't learn how to treat his problem. ED doesn't make George less of a person. His health

care team is there to help improve his quality of life. They are professionals and are not permitted to discuss his personal issues with anyone else without his permission. Knowing this could help George open up.

2. **George expects his doctor to ask about his ED.**
   Possible solution: As we discussed above, that may not happen. George should assume that he has to bring up the topic and choose a way to make it happen.

3. **George misses an opportunity to use the nurse to convey his need to talk to the doctor.**
   Possible solution: There are many ways to get the doctor's attention. This way would have worked. He must now try a different approach.

4. **Dr. Neverlisten is distracted by phone calls.**
   Possible solution: George deserves the doctor's undivided attention and should ask Dr. Neverlisten to focus on him. This can be done in a non-confrontational way. He can remind the doctor that he has important issues that he wants to review before he leaves.

5. **Dr. Neverlisten never asks George if he has any questions.**
   Possible solution: George must bring up the topic. He should write his questions down and prepare to have this discussion, as suggested above.

6. **George doesn't mention his ED.**
   Possible solution: He can make another appointment, call his doctor and discuss it over the phone, or plan to bring it up at the next regular visit. He can always ask for help. His wife could help and bring it up instead of him. It can be very helpful to have your partner participate in the discussion, especially because he or she should understand your needs and assist with any treatment that you choose.

7. **Dr. Neverlisten never improves.**
   Possible solution: If you have tried repeatedly to communicate with your doctor (or other health care provider) and have not seen any improvement, it may be time to find a different one.

Don't let your personal discomfort with a topic, or your health care provider's hesitancy to talk, keep you from getting the help that you need. Mention your concerns today.

FOR YOU AND YOUR PARTNER

1 How would you have responded to the encounter with Dr. Neverlisten?

2 Has this ever happened to you? How did you respond?

3 How will you prepare for your next visit with a health care professional?

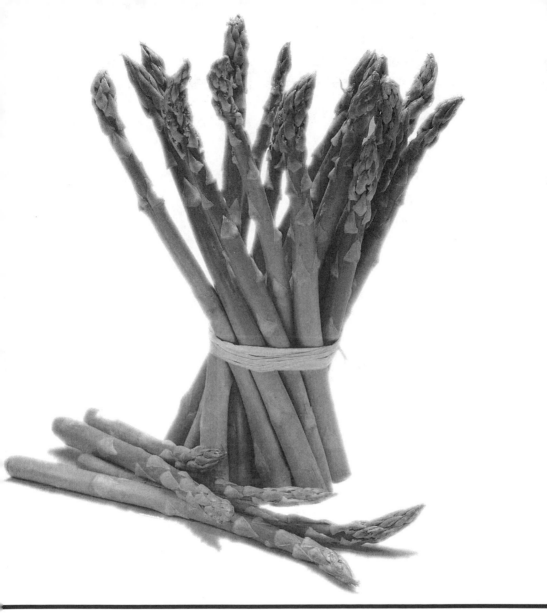

Chapter 11
Recipes for Love

Here are several recipes that use some of the aphrodisiacs listed in chapter 6. All come from cookbooks published by the American Diabetes Association: The aphrodisiac ingredients are marked with an asterisk (*).

APPETIZERS AND BEVERAGES

CHICKEN DRUMSTICKS
From *Healthy Calendar Diabetic Cooking*
Number of Servings: 6 ∎ Serving Size: 2 drumsticks

Ingredients
1 medium onion, chopped
2 garlic* cloves, sliced
¼ cup red wine* vinegar
Dijon mustard*
1 Tbsp olive* oil
½ tsp salt (optional)
¼ tsp ground black pepper
12 chicken legs, skinned
2 cups dry bread crumbs

Directions
1. Preheat oven to 350 degrees F.
2. In a blender or food processor, puree onion, garlic, vinegar, mustard, olive oil, salt, and pepper.
3. In a large bowl, add drumsticks and cover with marinade, turning to coat. Cover and refrigerate for 15 minutes.
4. Remove drumsticks from marinade and roll in bread crumbs, coating well.
5. Arrange drumsticks in the bottom of a shallow baking dish. Bake for 25–30 minutes or until done.

Exchanges Per Serving: 1 ½ Starch, 3 Lean Meat
Nutrition Information: Calories 280; Calories From Fat 75; Total Fat 8 g; Saturated Fat 1 g; Cholesterol 77 mg; Sodium 391 mg; Total Carbohydrate 21 g; Dietary Fiber 1 g; Sugars 3 g; Protein 28 g.

CHOCOLATE ALMOND COFFEE
From *Brand-Name Diabetic Meals in Minutes*
Number of Servings: 1 ∎ Serving Size: 1 cup

Ingredients
1 cup strongly brewed hot coffee
1 Tbsp Equal
2 tsp unsweetened cocoa* powder
¼ tsp almond* extract

Directions
Combine all ingredients in beverage mug until blended. Serve immediately.

Exchanges Per Serving: Free Food
Nutrition Information: Calories 19; Calories From Fat 0; Total Fat 1 g; Saturated Fat 0 g; Cholesterol 0 mg; Sodium 5 mg; Total Carbohydrate 3 g; Dietary Fiber 0 g; Sugars 0 g; Protein 0 g.

BREAKFAST AND BRUNCH

CHILLED MELON AND BERRY NECTAR

From *More Diabetic Meals in 30 Minutes—Or Less*
Number of Servings: 6 ∎ Serving Size: ½ cup

Ingredients

1 cup cantaloupe chunks
1 cup honeydew chunks
¼ cup dry white wine*
2 Tbsp orange juice
2 Tbsp sugar
1 cup buttermilk, low-fat
1 cup blueberries

Directions

In a food processor or blender, combine the melons, wine, juice, and
sugar. Puree until almost smooth. Add the buttermilk and process again.
Top each serving with blueberries.

Exchanges Per Serving: 1 Fruit
Nutrition Information: Calories 67; Calories From Fat 5; Total Fat 1 g; Saturated Fat
0 g; Cholesterol 1 mg; Sodium 49 mg; Total Carbohydrate 13 g; Dietary Fiber 1 g;
Sugars 12 g; Protein 2 g.

FRESH HERB OMELET

From *More Diabetic Meals in 30 Minutes—Or Less*
Number of Servings: 6 ▌ Serving Size: ⅙ of recipe

Ingredients

1 Tbsp olive* oil
1 cup red pepper, diced
1 cup fresh mushrooms, sliced
1 cup scallions, sliced
2 cloves garlic,* minced
4 slices whole-wheat bread, crusts removed (3 oz total)
1 cup low-fat cottage cheese
4 eggs
8 egg whites
¾ cup evaporated (fat-free) skim milk
1 Tbsp fresh basil,* minced
1 Tbsp fresh rosemary, minced
2 tsp fresh chives, minced
1 Tbsp fresh parsley,* minced
1 pinch fresh ground pepper and salt to taste

Directions

1. Preheat the oven to 350 degrees F. Heat the oil in a skillet over medium high heat. Sauté the pepper, mushrooms, and scallions for 6 minutes. Add the garlic and sauté for 3 more minutes.
2. Place the bread slices in a large casserole dish. Combine the remaining ingredients and pour the egg mixture on top of the bread. Add the cooked vegetables. Bake for about 25–40 minutes until the omelet is slightly puffed and set.

Exchanges Per Serving: 1 Starch, 1 Vegetable, 2 Lean Meat
Nutrition Information: Calories 222; Calories From Fat 62; Total Fat 7 g; Saturated Fat 2 g; Cholesterol 144 mg; Sodium 483 mg; Total Carbohydrate 18 g; Dietary Fiber 2 g; Sugars 8 g; Protein 22 g.

YOGURT WITH PEACH PUREE AND FRESH RASPBERRIES

From *Cooking with the Diabetic Chef*
Number of Servings 4 ∎ Serving Size: 9 oz

Ingredients
8 oz canned sliced peaches
8 oz fresh raspberries*
16 oz low-fat vanilla yogurt
1 cup walnuts, roughly chopped
4 fresh mint leaves

Directions
1. Drain the peaches and puree them in a blender or food processor until smooth. Wash the raspberries.
2. In a small bowl, place ⅛ of the yogurt at the bottom. Place ⅛ of the peach puree on top. Place ⅛ of the raspberries on the peach layer. Repeat this layer and then top with chopped walnuts. Garnish each glass with a few raspberries and a mint leaf.

Exchanges Per Serving: ½ Milk, 1 Fruit, 3 ½ Fat
Nutrition Information: Calories 297; Calories From Fat 163; Total Fat 18 g; Saturated Fat 2 g; Cholesterol 7 mg; Sodium 83 mg; Total Carbohydrate 25 g; Dietary Fiber 6 g; Sugars 17 g; Protein 14 g.

DIPS, SAUCES, AND CONDIMENTS

GUACAMOLE

From *The Complete Quick and Hearty Diabetic Cookbook*
Number of Servings: 8 ∎ Serving Size: ¼ cup

Ingredients

2 large ripe avocados,* peeled, pit removed, and mashed
½ chopped onion
2 jalapeno peppers, seeds removed, finely chopped
2 Tbsp minced fresh parsley*
2 Tbsp lime juice
⅛ tsp fresh ground black pepper
2 medium tomatoes, finely chopped
1 medium clove garlic,* minced
1 Tbsp olive* oil
½ tsp salt

Directions

In a large mixing bowl, combine all ingredients, blending well. Cover and refrigerate for at least one to two hours.

Exchanges Per Serving: 1 Vegetable, 2 ½ Fat
Nutrition Information: Calories 132; Calories From Fat 102; Total Fat 11 g; Saturated Fat 2 g; Cholesterol 0 mg; Sodium 146 mg; Total Carbohydrate 9 g; Dietary Fiber 5 g; Sugars 3 g; Protein 2 g.

NUOM CHUC SAUCE

From *Quick & Easy Diabetic Recipes for One*
Number of Servings: 4 ■ Serving Size: 2 Tablespoons

Prepare this sauce two hours before serving for the best flavor. The leftover sauce will stay stored in the refrigerator in a covered glass container for one week.

Ingredients

1 Tbsp rice wine* vinegar
1 Tbsp lime juice
2 Tbsp prepared fish sauce
2 Tbsp water
1 Tbsp sugar
1 tsp dry white wine*
1 clove garlic,* minced
¼ tsp cayenne pepper
1 Tbsp finely julienned carrots*
1 Tbsp finely julienned green onion

Directions

Combine all the ingredients in a small, non-plastic bowl and stir until the sugar dissolves.

Exchanges Per Serving: ½ Carbohydrate
Nutrition Information: Calories 24; Calories From Fat 0; Total Fat 0 g; Saturated Fat 0 g; Cholesterol 0 mg; Sodium 316 mg; Total Carbohydrate 6 g; Dietary Fiber 0 g; Sugars 5 g; Protein 1 g.

ENTREES

CHICKEN SATAY

From *More Diabetic Meals in 30 Minutes—Or Less*
Number of Servings: 6 ∎ Serving Size: about 3–4 oz

A satay is a spicy Indian kabob.

Ingredients

1 Tbsp corn oil
3 Tbsp lime juice
3 garlic cloves*
1 red chili, minced
1 Tbsp honey*
1 tsp ground coriander seeds*
1 ½ lb boneless, skinless chicken breasts, cubed into 1-inch pieces

Directions

1. In a blender, combine all ingredients for the sauce. Place the chicken cubes in a bowl, cover with the sauce, and marinate in a refrigerator for four hours. Prepare an outside grill with an oiled rack set 4 inches above the heat source. On a gas grill, set the heat to high.
2. If using wooden kabob skewers, soak six of them in warm water for 15 minutes. This prevents the skewers from catching on fire while the kabobs cook. Then thread the chicken cubes on the skewers. Grill the satays for about 4–5 minutes total, until the chicken is cooked through.

Exchanges Per Serving: 4 Very Lean Meat, ½ Fat
Nutrition Information per serving: Calories 162; Calories From Fat 43; Total Fat 5 g; Saturated Fat 1 g; Cholesterol 69 mg; Sodium 60 mg; Total Carbohydrate 3 g; Dietary Fiber 0 g; Sugars 3 g; Protein 25 g.

MARINATED LAMB CHOPS

From *More Diabetic Meals in 30 Minutes–Or Less*
Number of Servings: 6 ∎ Serving Size: 3 oz

Ingredients

½ cup dry red wine*
¼ cup raspberry* vinegar
2 Tbsp Dijon mustard*
1 pinch fresh ground pepper and salt to taste
2 lb lamb chops

Directions

Combine the first four ingredients. Add the lamb chops and marinate in
the refrigerator for one to two hours. Grill or broil the lamb chops until
done as desired.

Exchanges Per Serving: 2 Lean Meat, ½ Fat
Nutrition Information per serving: Calories 135; Calories From Fat 58; Total Fat
6 g; Saturated Fat 2 g; Cholesterol 56 mg; Sodium 86 mg; Total Carbohydrate 1 g;
Dietary Fiber 0 g; Sugars 1 g; Protein 17 g.

SOUPS

CARROT AND GINGER SOUP
From *Cooking with the Diabetic Chef*
Number of Servings: 4 ■ Serving Size: 1/2 cup

Ingredients
½ Tbsp olive* oil
½ cup shallots, chopped
4 Tbsp ginger,* minced
1 ½ lb carrots,* diced
1 quart low-fat, low-sodium chicken broth
1 dash white pepper
4 Tbsp heavy cream
1 Tbsp fresh chives, chopped

Directions
1. In a large pot, heat the olive oil over medium heat. Add the shallots and ginger. Cook until the shallots become translucent. Add the diced carrots and enough chicken stock to cover them. Bring the liquid to a boil then reduce the heat to simmer. Skim off any scum or fat which floats to the surface, cover the pot tightly, and cook for 15–20 minutes, or until the carrots are very soft.
2. Place the carrots and chicken stock into a blender or food processor and puree until smooth. Season with salt and white pepper. Serve immediately and garnish with a dollop of heavy cream and fresh chives.

Exchanges Per Serving: 4 Vegetable
Nutrition Information: Calories 105; Calories From Fat 19; Total Fat 2 g; Saturated Fat 1 g; Cholesterol 0 mg; Sodium 353 mg; Total Carbohydrate 21 g; Dietary Fiber 5 g; Sugars 12 g; Protein 2 g.

TORTELLINI SOUP

From *Healthy Calendar Diabetic Cooking*
Number of Servings: 7 ∎ Serving Size: 1 cup

Ingredients

Cooking spray
2 cups reduced-fat or lean Italian turkey sausage, crumbled
½ cup finely diced onion
¼ cup red wine*
½ Tbsp dried basil*
½ Tbsp dried oregano
1 15-oz can no-salt added diced tomatoes with juice
3 14.5-oz cans fat-free reduced sodium chicken broth
2 ½ cups uncooked three-cheese tortellini
½ tsp ground black pepper

Directions

1. Coat a large soup pot with cooking spray. Add sausage and onion and cook over medium-high heat for seven minutes or until sausage begins to brown.
2. Add wine to deglaze pan. Cook for two minutes or until wine is almost completely evaporated.
3. Add basil and oregano and cook for one minute. Add tomatoes and broth. Bring to a boil, then reduce heat and simmer for five minutes.
4. Add tortellini and pepper. Cook for another 10 minutes.

Exchanges Per Serving: 1 Starch, 2 Lean Meat, 1 Vegetable
Nutrition Information: Calories 216; Calories From Fat 63; Total Fat 7 g; Saturated Fat 2 g; Cholesterol 43 mg; Sodium 858 mg; Total Carbohydrate 23 g; Dietary Fiber 2 g; Sugars 5 g; Protein 16 g.

BREADS

BANANA GINGER MUFFINS

From *More Diabetic Meals in 30 Minutes–Or Less*
Number of Servings: 12 ∎ Serving Size: 1 muffin

Grating real ginger into these muffins is the secret to their flavor.

Ingredients

1 ½ cups white flour
1 cup whole-wheat flour
2 tsp baking powder
1 tsp cinnamon
1 egg white
1 cup milk, fat-free (skim)
¼ cup applesauce, unsweetened
2 Tbsp canola oil
2 Tbsp brown sugar
2 bananas,* mashed
2 tsp ginger,* grated fresh

Directions

1. Preheat oven to 350 degrees. Combine the flours, baking powder, and cinnamon in a medium bowl. In a large bowl, combine the remaining ingredients and mix well. Slowly add the dry ingredients to the large bowl and mix until blended. Do not overbeat.
2. Pour the batter into 12 nonstick muffin cups and bake for 20–25 minutes. Remove muffins from oven and let cool slightly. Remove muffins from pan and let cool completely.

Exchanges Per Serving: 2 Carbohydrates
Nutrition Information: Calories 156; Calories From Fat 29; Total Fat 3 g; Saturated Fat 0 g; Cholesterol 18 mg; Sodium 83 mg; Total Carbohydrate 28 g; Dietary Fiber 2 g; Sugars 7 g; Protein 5 g.

GARLIC BREAD

From *Forbidden Foods Diabetic Cooking*
Number of Servings: 12 ∎ Serving Size: 2 slices

For a delightful variation that goes well with roasted pork or turkey, substitute crumbled, dry sage leaves for the oregano.

Ingredients

4 Tbsp extra-virgin olive* oil
2 Tbsp unsalted margarine or butter, melted
2 garlic cloves,* minced
½ tsp dried oregano
¼ tsp seasoned salt
1 (1 lb) loaf Italian or French bread, cut into 24 ½-inch slices

Directions

1. Preheat the oven to 400 degrees F.
2. In a small bowl, combine the oil, butter, garlic, oregano, and salt. Brush the mixture on one side of each bread slice then press the slices back together to form a loaf. Wrap the loaf in foil and bake until hot in the center, 15–20 minutes.

Exchanges Per Serving: 1 ½ Starch, 1 Fat
Nutrition Information: Calories 148; Calories From Fat 58; Total Fat 6 g; Saturated Fat 1 g; Cholesterol 0 mg; Sodium 258 mg; Total Carbohydrate 19 g; Dietary Fiber 1 g; Sugars 0 g; Protein 4 g.

VEGETABLES

ASPARAGUS SOUFFLE
From *Flavorful Seasons Cookbook*
Number of Servings: 6 ∎ Serving Size: 1 cup

Ingredients
2 ½ lb fresh asparagus,* trimmed and cut into 1-inch pieces
1 egg, beaten
1 cup grated low-fat Swiss cheese
1 cup diced cooked low-fat turkey bacon
2 tsp canola oil
2 Tbsp Parmesan cheese
1 Tbsp cornstarch or arrowroot powder
¼ cup low-fat, low-sodium chicken broth
2 egg whites, beaten until stiff

Directions
1. Preheat the oven to 350 degrees.
2. Steam the asparagus in a metal steamer over boiling water for five to six minutes. Drain.
3. Combine the asparagus with the egg, Swiss cheese, turkey bacon, oil, and Parmesan cheese.
4. Combine the cornstarch or arrowroot powder with the chicken broth and stir until smooth. Add to the asparagus mixture.
5. Fold in the beaten egg whites until they disappear.
6. Pour the mixture into a greased soufflé dish and bake for 25–30 minutes until puffed and firm.

Exchanges Per Serving: 2 Lean Meat, 1 Vegetable, ½ Fat
Nutrition Information: Calories 154; Calories From Fat 79; Total Fat 9 g; Saturated Fat 3 g; Cholesterol 89 mg; Sodium 351 mg; Total Carbohydrate 5 g; Dietary Fiber 2 g; Sugars 2 g; Protein 15 g.

COLLARD GREENS

From *The New Soul Food Cookbook for People with Diabetes*
Number of Servings: 8 ∎ Serving Size: 1 cup

Ingredients

4 lb collard greens
3 cups low-fat, low-sodium chicken broth
2 onions, chopped
3 cloves garlic,* crushed
1 tsp crushed red pepper flakes
1 tsp pepper

Directions

1. Wash and cut the collard greens and place them in a large stockpot. Add the remaining ingredients and enough water to cover.
2. Cook until tender, stirring occasionally, about 3 ½ hours. The flavors will blend even more if you let the greens sit for a bit after cooking.

Exchanges Per Serving: 3 Vegetable
Nutrition Information per serving: Calories 78; Calories From Fat 4; Total Fat 0 g; Saturated Fat 0 g; Cholesterol 0 mg; Sodium 240 mg; Total Carbohydrate 16 g; Dietary Fiber 6 g; Sugars 3 g; Protein 4 g.

DESSERTS

LINDA'S CHOCOLATE LOG
From *The Healthy HomeStyle Cookbook*
Number of Servings: 8 ▌ Serving Size: 1 slice

A jelly roll pan is the same as a cookie pan with edges that stand up on all four sides. Some cookie pans have one end open so cookies can slide off the pan.

Ingredients
1 banana* fresh or frozen, thawed
2 slices bread, white or wheat, cubed
2 chocolate* milk shake mixes (.75 oz)
½ cup egg substitute
½ tsp cream of tartar
½ tsp baking soda
1 tsp vanilla
½ cup low-fat ricotta cheese
1 tsp vanilla
4 artificial sweetener, packets

Directions
1. Combine cake ingredients in a blender or food processor and blend until smooth.
2. Spray jelly roll pan with nonstick cooking spray. Pour mixture into pan and spread to corners. Cook at 350 degrees F for 10 minutes.
3. Let stand one to two minutes. Remove from pan and cool. Prepare filling. These are the last three ingredients.
4. Blend filling ingredients. Spread on cake and roll up.
5. Wrap in foil and refrigerate or cut in slices and serve immediately. Serve on dessert plates plain or topped with sliced fruit or a fruit sauce.

Exchanges Per Serving: 1 Carbohydrate
Nutrition Information per serving: Calories 62; Calories From Fat 18; Total Fat 2 g; Saturated Fat 1 g; Cholesterol 5 mg; Sodium 178 mg; Total Carbohydrate 11 g; Dietary Fiber 1 g; Protein 4 g.

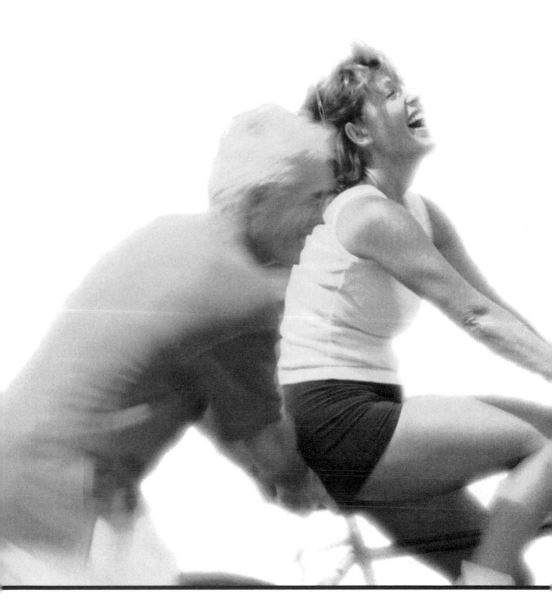

Chapter 12
Resources

Here are some resources for you, your partner, and your health professional to use in your search for reliable information about diabetes and diabetes-related sexual complications.

DVD

Sex, Intimacy, and Diabetes. This entertaining and informative 30-minute DVD provides a frank discussion of relationship and physical intimacy issues that individuals with diabetes and their partners face. Produced by dLifeTV. Available from the Public Health Foundation Learning Resource Center at *www.phf.org* or call 1-877-252-1200.

PUBLICATIONS

Everything Men with Diabetes Want to Know But Are Afraid to Ask: New Perspectives on Erectile Dysfunction. Chicago, American Association of Diabetes Educators, 1999.

PDR for Nutritional Supplements. Montvale, NJ, Thomson PDR, 2001.

Duke, James A. *The Green Pharmacy Herbal Handbook.* New York, Rodale Reach, 2000.

Love, Susan. *Dr. Susan Love's Menopause & Hormone Book.* New York, Three Rivers Press, 2003.

Polonsky, William H. *Diabetes Burnout.* Alexandria, VA, American Diabetes Association, 1999.

Rice, Donna, Bob Rice. *Diabetes and Erectile Dysfunction—A Quick 'n' Easy Handbook for the Diabetes Educator.* Brighton, MI, Bella Vista Publications.

Roszler, Janis. *Diabetes on Your OWN Terms.* New York, Marlowe & Company, 2007.

Roszler, J. Appendix C: Use of herbs, supplements, and alternative therapies. *American Dietetic Association Guide to Diabetes Medical Nutrition Therapy and Education.* Chicago, American Dietetic Association, 2005.

Roszler, Janis, William H. Polonsky, and Steven V Edelman.
The Secrets of Living and Loving with Diabetes. Chicago, Surrey Books,
2004.

Rubin, Alan L. *Diabetes for Dummies, 2nd Edition.* Indianapolis, IN,
Wiley Publishing, 2004.

WEBSITES

www.aace.com
The official site of the American Association of Clinical
Endocrinologists.

www.aasect.org
This is the official site of the American Association of Sex
Educators, Counselors, and Therapists. It can help you locate
a counselor in your area.

www.americanheart.org
The official site of the American Heart Association.

www.breastimplantsafety.org
This website offers unbiased, science-based information on breast
implant options that is written by some of the leading plastic
surgeons in the country.

www.calorieking.com
This website contains nutrient listings of many common foods. Check
here to locate the carbohydrate, fat, or sodium content of a particular
food item.

www.cartoonmd.com
This site, created by endocrinologist Justin Grady Matrisciano, MD,
uses cartoons and animated videos to explain the action of diabetes
medications and other diabetes-related concepts.

www.caverject.com
  This site provides information about Caverject, an injected ED medication.

www.cfsan.fda.gov/~dms/ds-warn.html
  The above website contains a list of dietary supplement ingredients for which the FDA has issued warnings.

www.consumeraffairs.com
  This website is an independent source of consumer news and recall information. It also provides forms that can be filled out with consumer-related complaints.

www.consumerlab.com
  An independent site that reviews the safety and effectiveness of herbs and supplements.

www.cialis.com
  This site provides information about sexual issues and Cialis medication.

www.dearjanis.com
  Personal website of Janis Roszler, RD, CDE, LD/N—contains an interactive message board, articles, podcasts, and radio show interviews.

www.diabeteseducator.org
  The official site of the American Association of Diabetes Educators—offers an educator locator service.

www.diabetes.org
  The official website of the American Diabetes Association.

www.dLife.com
  The official website of dLifeTV program on CNBC.

www.diabetes.niddk.nih.gov
This is the site of the National Diabetes Information Clearinghouse, run by the National Institute of Diabetes and Digestive and Kidney Diseases and National Institutes of Health (NIH).

www.eatright.org
The official site of the American Dietetic Association.

www.erectile-dysfunction-treatment.org
Website of the Erectile Dysfunction Information Center.

www.fda.gov/buyonlineguide
Link to the FDA online guide: "Buying Prescription Medicines Online: A Consumer Safety Guide."

www.fda.gov/oc/buyonline/buyonlineform.htm
Use the above link to report problems that don't involve a serious or life-threatening reaction. To report false claims to the Federal Trade Commission, call (877) 382-4357.

www.fda.gov/counterfeit/
A link to the FDA report on combating counterfeit drugs.

www.fda.gov/medwatch
Report negative medical effects at this site.

www.fda.gov/oc/enforcement.html
This website lists enforcement actions that have been taken against the promoters of different products.

www.hisandherhealth.com
A website that provides information about sexual issues.

www.levitra.com
This website provides information about sexual issues and Levitra medication.

www.medlineplus.gov
This site provides information about medications and medical conditions. Sponsored by the U.S. National Library of Medicine and NIH.

www.nwcr.ws
The National Weight Control Registry (NWCR).

www.phf.org
This is the official website of the Public Health Foundation.

www.plasticsurgery.org
This is the official website of the American Society of Plastic Surgeons.

www.quackwatch.com
Provides a guide to medical misinformation and health fraud. Check out Internet health-related rumors at this site.

www.rejoyn.com
Website that sells ED products.

www.safeoysters.org
A site that offers information about the vibrio vulnificus infection that can develop in people with diabetes and other medical conditions after consuming improperly cooked shellfish.

www.snopes.com
Debunks internet rumors of all types.

www.timmmedical.com
A source of ED treatment products.

www.togetherrxaccess.com
This site offers prescription assistance. Call 1-800-444-4106 for additional information.

www.urbanlegends.about.com
An additional site that debunks Internet rumors.

www.urologyhealth.org
A patient education site written and reviewed by urology experts in partnership with the American Urological Association Foundation.

www.viagra.com
This website provides information about sexual issues and Viagra medication.

www.vivus.com
A source of ED treatment products.

www.webcomplaints@ora.fda.gov
Report emails or websites that promote illegal medical products to this site.

www.webmd.com
A reliable source of medical information of all types, including sexual issues.

www.yogafinder.com
This site contains an extensive yoga directory that offers information about classes and teachers in your area.

www.yogajournal.com
This site offers articles, workout guidance, and step-by-step instruction in the art of yoga.

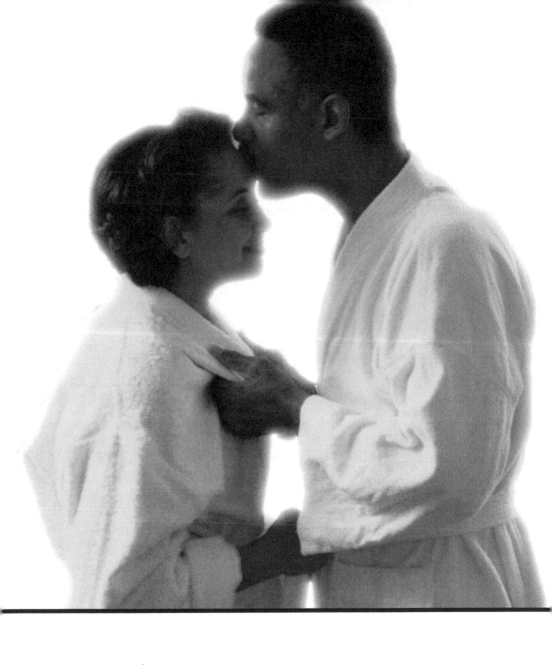

Appendix

PRESCRIPTION ASSISTANCE PROGRAMS

The following pharmaceutical companies have prescription assistance programs.

Pharmaceutical Companies	Name of Program	Contact Information
3M Pharmaceuticals	3M Pharmaceuticals Patient Assistance Programs	275-6W-13 St. Paul, MN 55144-1000 1-800-328-0255 *www.mmm.com*
Abbott Laboratories	Abbott Laboratories Patient Assistant Programs	200 Abbott Park Road, D-31C, J23 Abbott Park, IL 60064 1-800-222-6885 *www.abbott.com*
Animas Corp. • Insulin Pump • Pump supplies	Diabetes Trust Fund (for children 21 and under with current health care coverage)	1-877-YES-PUMP (937-7867) Anne Barton, x1149
AstraZeneca	AstraZeneca Foundation Patient Assistance Program	P.O. Box 15197 Wilmington, DE 19850 1-800-424-3727 *www.astrazeneca-us.com*
Sanofi-Aventis Pharmaceuticals, Inc. • Amaryl (glimepiride) • Lantus (insulin)	Lovenox Patient Assistance Program Aventis Patient Assistance Program	2211 Sanders Road NTB7 Northbrook, IL 60067 1-888-632-8607; 1-888-875-9951 *www.aventis.com*
Bayer Corporation • Precose (acarbose)	Bayer Patient Assistance Program	P.O. Box 29209 Phoenix, AZ 85038-9209 1-800-998-9180 *www.bayer.com*

BD (Becton, Dickinson and Company)	BD Diabetes	1 Becton Drive Franklin Lakes, NJ 07417 888-232-2737 *http://www.bddiabetes.com/us/*
Bristol-Myers Squibb Company • Glucophage (metformin hydrocloride) • Glucovance	Bristol-Myers Squibb Patient Assistance Foundation, Inc.	P.O. Box 52001 Phoenix, AZ 85072-9160 1-800-736-0003 *www.bms.com*
Eli Lilly • Humulin (insulin) • Humalog (insulin) • Glucagon (emergency kit)	Lilly Cares (under 65 and not on Medicare) Lilly Answers (for seniors)	Lilly Cares Temporary Prescription Assistance Program P.O. Box 230999 Centreville, VA 20120 800-545-6962 *www.lillydiabetes.com* Lilly Answers 877-795-4559 *www.lillyanswers.com*
GlaxoSmithKline • Avandia (rosiglitazone) • Avandimet (combo of Metformin and Avandia)	GlaxoWellcome Patient Assistance Program SmithKline Foundation Access to Care	P.O. Box 2564 Maryland Heights, MO 63043-8564 1-800-546-0420; 1-800-729-4544 *www.ipp.gsk.com*
Medtronic Mini-Med • Insulin pumps • Pump supplies	Mini-Med Financial Assistance Program	1-800-MINI-MED
Merck and Co., Inc.	The Merck Patient Assistance Program	One Merck Drive P.O. Box 100 Whitehouse Station, NJ 08889-0100 1-908-423-1000 Hours: 8:30am–5:30pm *www.merck.com*

Pharmaceutical Companies	Name of Program	Contact Information
Novartis • Starlix	Novartis Pharmaceuticals Corporation Patient Program Assistance	P.O. Box 66556 St. Louis, MO 63166-6556 1-800-277-2254 *www.novartis.com*
Novo Nordisk • Pharmaceuticals, Inc. • Prandin (repaglinide) • Novolin (insulin) • Novolog (insulin)	Patient Assistance Program (Insulin Products) Indigent Program Administrator (Prandin)	100 College Road West Princeton, NJ 08540 800-727-6500 100 Overlook Ctr, Ste 200 Princeton, NJ 08540 1-800-727-6500
Pfizer • Glucotrol (glipizide) • Glucotrol XL (glipizide–extended release) • Diabinese (chlorpropamide) • Glucamide • Metaglip (combo of Metformin and Glipizide)	Connection to Care	P.O. Box 66585 St. Louis, MO 63166 1-800-707-8990 *www.pfizer.com*
Pharmacia - *SUBSIDIARY OF PFIZER* • Glyset (miglitol) • Micronase (glyburide) • Tolinase • Orinase • DiaBeta	Please contact Pfizer for information on assistance programs	P.O. Box 66585 St. Louis, MO 63166 1-800-707-8990 *www.pfizer.com*
Procter and Gamble Pharmaceuticals	Procter and Gamble Pharmaceuticals Patient Assistance Program	P.O. Box 5663 St. Louis, MO 63166-6553 1-800-830-9049 *www.pgpharma.com*
Roche Laboratories Inc.	Roche Laboratories Patient Assistance Program	340 Kingsland Street Nutley, NJ 07110 1-800-285-4484 *www.rocheusa.com*

Takeda Pharmaceuticals North America • Actos (pioglitazone hydrochloride)	Takeda Patient Assistance Program	P.O. Box 66552 St. Louis, MO 63166 1-800-830-9159 *www.takedapharm.com*
TogetherRX Access	Provides some diabetes medications and blood glucose meters and strips at a reduced price	1-800-444-4106 *www.togetherrxaccess. com*
Veteran's Administration	For active and retired military personnel and their families	1-877-222-8387 or *www.va.gov* or *www.tricare.osd.mil/* (mail order pharmacy)

www.diabetes.org

MEDICATIONS THAT CAN INTERFERE WITH ED MEDICATIONS

The following medications may cause ED medications to act in an unexpected way and/or last longer than desired. Please review your use of these medicines with your health care team as well:

Antibiotic/Antifungal
Biaxin (clarithromycin)
Clotrimazole
Erythromycin
Diflucan
Sporanox
Ketoconazole
Miconazole
Noroxin

Cardiovascular
Amiodarone (Cordarone)
Norvasc

Digitoxin
Diltiazem
Disopyramide (Norpace)
Plendil (felodipine)
DynaCirc (isradipine)
Cozaar (losartan)
Nifedipine
Quinidine
Verapamil
Norvasc
Cardizem
Cardizem–SR
Cardizem–CD
Procardia
Procardia–XL
Adalat CC
Calan
Calan–SR
Isoptin
Isoptin–SR
Covera–HS

Cholesterol lowering
Lipitor (atorvastatin)
Mevacor
Zocor (simvastin)

Central nervous system
Alprazolam (Xanax)
Carbamazepine (Tegretol)
Prozac (fluoxetine)
Luvox (fluvoxamine)
Imipramine (Tofranil)
Serzone (nefazodone)
Phenobarbital
Phenytoin (Dilantin)

Zoloft
Triazolam (Halcion)

Other
Acetaminophen
Hismanal (astemizole)
Tagamet (cimetidine)
Propulsid (cisapride)
Cyclosporine
Dexamethasone (Decadron/Hexadrol)

Although these pills relax the muscles and dilate blood vessels so that blood can flow to the penis, each is slightly different. If one brand does not work after several attempts, adjust the strength (with a doctor's guidance) or try a different brand. You can also use a pill along with a vacuum pump or suppository if desired.

MEDICATIONS THAT MAY ENCOURAGE DEVELOPMENT OF ED PROBLEMS

The following is a partial list of medications that may encourage the development of erection problems. The list is taken from *Healthwise* (2004).

For High Blood Pressure
Norvasc (amlodipine)
Tenormin (atenolol)
Catapres (clonidine)
Aldomet (methyldopa)
Lopressor, Toprol XL (metoprolol)
Adalat, Adalat CC, Procardia (nifedipine)
Inderal (propranolol)

Diuretics
Diamox (acetazolamide)

Diuril (chlorothiazide)
Hygroton, Thalitone (chlorthalidone)
Apresoline (hydralazine)
Lopressor HCT (hydrochlorothiazide and metoprolol)
Aldactone, Spironol (spironolactone)
Dyrenium (tramterene)

Antidepressants
Elavil, Endep, Vanatrip (Amitriptyline)
Celexa (Citalopram)
Lexapro (Escitalopram oxalate)
Prozac, Sarafem (Fluoxetine)
Luvox (Fluvoxamine)
Tofranil (Imipramine)
Marplan (Isocarboxazid)
Aventyl HCl, Pamelor (Nortriptyline hydrochloride)
Paxil (Paroxetine)
Nardil (Phenelzine)
Zoloft (Sertraline)
Parnate (Tranylcypromine)

Cholesterol lowering
Lopid (Gemfibrozil)
Nicolar, Nicotinex (Niacin)

Cardiovascular
Lanoxicaps, Lanoxin (Digoxin)

Index

A

AADE-7 self care behaviors, 147–151
  being active, 148–149
  healthy coping, 151
  healthy eating, 148
  monitoring, 149
  problem solving, 150
  reducing risks, 151
  taking medications, 149

Abstention, to heighten desire, 92–93

ACE inhibitors, 48

Acidophilus, 84

A1C levels
  glucose equivalents, 46
  goals for, 45
  for pregnancy, 85

Actra-Rx, 125

Aging, 135–152
  dating and, 144
  diabetes care and, 140.
    See also AADE-7 self care behaviors
  HIV/AIDS in elderly, 144
  intimacy and, 146–147, 152
  normal effects of, 136–146
    bad breath, 139
    diabetes symptoms vs., 138–139
    hearing loss, 140
    heart problems, 143–144
    for men, 138
    new relationships, 144–145
    partner, loss of, 144
    physical appearance, disliking,
      145–146
    sleep changes, 139–140
    urinary incontinence, 140–142
    for women, 137–138
  personal sexual gratification, 145
  widower's syndrome, 144

Alcoholic beverages, 74. *See also* Wine

Almonds, 100, 165

Alpha-blockers, 58

American Association of Diabetes
  Educators, 147
  self care behaviors. *See* AADE-7
    self care behaviors
  website address, 184

American Association of Sex Educators,
  Counselors, and Therapists, 26, 68

American Diabetes Association
  advocacy department, 21
  alcohol intake, 74
  blood glucose goals, 45–46
  blood lipid goals, 49
  carbohydrate intake, 43, 77
  website address, 184

American Dietetic Association, 40

American Heart Association, 143, 183

American Society of Plastic Surgeons,
  130

Anger, 26–27, 151

Animal aphrodisiac myths, 131

Aniseed, 100

Antibiotics, 85, 193

Antidepressants, 76, 196

Aphrodisiacs, 99–103
  Bremelanotide, 103
  foods, 100–102. *See also* Recipes
  myths, 131
  placebos, 99–100, 102
  scams, 130–131

Appendix, 189–196

ARBs (angiotensin receptor blockers), 48

Arginine, 107

Aromatherapy, 94–96. *See also* Scents

Ashtanga yoga, 22

Ashwaganda, 107

Asparagus, 102, 177

Autonomic neuropathy, 23

Avocado, 102, 169

B

Bad breath, 139

Bananas, 102, 175, 179

Basil, 100, 167, 174

Belly dancing, 145

Beta blockers, 48

Birth control, 85, 86

Bladder infections, 83–85

Blame, 116, 117

Blood glucose levels
    cayenne extract and, 127
    depression and, 19
    fatigue and, 76
    ginseng and, 109
    goals for, 45–46
    intimacy and, 73–75
    libido and, 30
    for sexual activity, 150

Blood glucose monitoring, 45–46, 149
    herbal supplements and, 106
    menopause and, 74
    menstruation and, 74
    prior to sexual activity, 73–74
    when eating out, 74

Blood pressure, 47–48
    ginseng and, 109
    medications for, 48, 195
    orgasm and, 80
    recommended level, 47

Breast augmentation, 129–130, 183

Breast enhancement scams, 128–129

Bremelanotide, 103

Bruising, 50

Butea superba, 108

Byetta, 41, 75

C

Calcium channel blockers, 48

Calories
    calculator for exercise, 97–98
    in foods, 183
    limiting severely, 77

Carbohydrates
    counting, 36–37
    healthy amounts of, 43, 77

Cardamom, 100

Cardiovascular medicine, 193–194, 196

Cardura, 58

Carnitine, 108

Carrots, 102, 173

Caverject, 60–61, 184

Cayenne extract, 126

Central nervous system medications, 194–195

Cervical caps, 86

Chocolate, 100, 165, 179

Cholesterol, 48–49

Cholesterol-lowering drugs, 194, 196

Cialis, 58–59, 184

Circulation problems, 47–49, 143–144

Cocoa, 165

Communication, 81, 111–122
  with doctors. *See* Doctors
  effective, tips for, 114–118
    blame, avoiding, 117
    discussion questions, 116
    emotions, sensitivity to,
      116–117
    fears, examining, 114–115
    follow-up, 118
    good things, focusing on, 117
    Jump Start Pledges, 122
    listening, 117
    patience, 118
    pillow talk, 118
    planning ahead, 116
    timing/location, 115
    topic, staying on, 117
    valuing discussion, 115
  embarrassment and, 113, 155–156,
    157
  hearing loss and, 140
  magic pencil technique, 119–122
  styles of
    embarrassment/
      miscommunication, 113
    passionate/open, 112–113
    secretive/distant, 114
Complications
  DVD about, 121
  misconceptions, 156–157
  reducing risk of, 151
  sexual, assessment quizzes, 8–11
Condoms, 86
Constriction rings, 63–64
Contraceptives. *See* Birth control
Coriander, 100, 171
Counseling
  for depression, 20

  for erectile dysfunction (ED), 68
  for relationship difficulties, 26
Country mallow, 108
Cranberry juice, 85
Creams
  for breast enhancement, 129
  for dry skin, 83

D

Dating, 28–29, 144–145
Dental hygiene, 139
Depression, 17–20, 151
  blood sugar levels and, 19
  counseling for, 20
  exercise and, 19
  marriage and, 17
  medications for, 20, 76
  physical effects of, 18
  risk assessment, 18–19
  spirituality and, 20
  testosterone and, 56
DHEA, 108
Diabetes
  complications. *See* Complications
  family risk factors, 86–87
  guilt about developing, 14–15
  keeping secret from partners, 28
  physical changes from, 33–51
    abnormal blood pressure, 47–48
    bruising, from injections, 50
    circulation problems, 47–49
    lipid levels, 48–49
    nerve damage (neuropathy), 44
    personal hygiene issues, 50
    weight gain, 34
  positive aspects of, 15, 16

positive attitude about, 29

type 2, 14

Diabetes care

AADE-7 self care. *See* AADE-7
self care behaviors

aging and, 140

blood glucose monitoring, 45–46

confidence in, 29

exhaustion from, 21

Diabetes classes, 121

Diabetes medications, 149

buying online, 185

erectile dysfunction (ED) and,
55

insulin, 34

low libido and, 75

prescription assistance programs,
31, 190–193

weight gain from, 34, 41

"Diabetes police," 26–27

Diaphragms, 85, 86

Dietitians, 40

Discrimination, job, 21

Diuretics, 48, 195–196

dLifeTV, 121, 184

Doctors

discussing depression with, 20

discussing sexual problems with,
153–162

appointments, extra time for,
157

communication problems/
solutions, 160–161

doctor's reluctance, assuming,
158, 161

doing research, 157–158

embarrassment and, 155–156,
157

erectile dysfunction, 154, 157,
158, 160–161

impediments to, 154–157

libido, 155

medical environment and, 154–155

nurses, help from, 159, 161

timing, 159

written questions/concerns, 159

DVDs

diabetes-related complications, 121

Sex, Intimacy and Diabetes, 182

E

Eating out, 36, 38, 74

ED. *See* Erectile dysfunction (ED)

Embarrassment, 113, 155–156, 157

Emotional intimacy, 2–3, 5–6

Emotions, 13–31, 151

anger, 26–27, 151

depression. *See* Depression

expressing, 15–16

financial pressures, 31

guilt, 14–16, 151

hopelessness, 156–157

rejection, fear of, 28–29

sexual interest, loss of, 30

stress. *See* Stress

Employment

job duties, adjusting, 21

loss of job, 31

rights and, 21

Endocrinologists, 158, 183

Erectile dysfunction (ED), 54–68

causes of

low testosterone, 55–56

medications, 55, 195–196

non-diabetes causes, 54

discussing with doctor, 154, 157, 158, 160–161
drug interactions, 58–59, 193–195
emotional response to, 116–117
prevalence of, 55
supplement scams, 125, 130
treatments for
    constriction rings, 63–64
    counseling, 68
    devices, 62–68
    herbal supplements, 106–110
    implants, 66–68
    injections, 60–61
    oral medications, 58–59, 193–195
    support sleeves, 65–66
    suppositories, 61–62
    testosterone, 56–58
    vacuum pumps, 64–65
Erectile Dysfunction Information Center, 185
Erotic media, 59, 92, 105
Estring, 143
Estrogen, 80, 143
Exercise, 43–44, 148–149
belly dancing, 145
benefits of, 146, 149
blood glucose levels and, 75
calorie calculator, 97–98
for depression, 19
for fatigue, 77
kegel exercises, 141–142
risks/recommendations, 23
safety, 23, 44, 73–74
sexual activity as, 73–74, 98, 149
sharing, 96–99
for stress reduction, 22
talk test, 44
walking, 98–99
weight training, 145–146
yoga, 22, 187

F

Fad diets, 77
Fatigue, 30, 76–79
from diabetes care, 21
sleep tips, 78
testosterone and, 56
Fats
blood lipids, 48–49
dietary, 48, 49
Fava beans, 100
Feelings. *See* Emotions
Fiber, 38–39
15/15 rule, 42
Figs, 102
Flomax, 58
Foreplay, 80, 81
4EVERON, 125
Fraudulent sexual products. *See* Sexual product scams
Friendships, 24

G

Garlic, 100, 164, 167, 169, 170, 171, 176, 178
Ginger, 101, 173, 175
Ginkgo biloba, 109, 126
Ginseng, 109
Guarana, 108
Guilt, 14–16, 151

H

Hatha yoga, 22

HDL cholesterol, 48–49

Hearing loss, 140

Heart attack, sexual activity following, 143–144

Herbal supplements, 106–110. *See also* individual herbs
dangerous, 125, 184
ED scams, 125, 130
libido enhancement scams, 130
penis enlargement scams, 126–127
safe use of, 106

Historic romances, 3, 4, 7

HIV/AIDS, 144

Honey, 101, 171

Hopelessness, 156–157

Hormones
estrogen, 80, 143
testosterone. *See* Testosterone

Horny goat weed extract, 126–127

Hypoglycemia
fatigue from, 77–78
15/15 rule, 42
weight gain and, 42

Hytrin, 58

I

Impotence. *See* Erectile dysfunction (ED)

Incontinence, 140–142

Insulin. *See also* Diabetes medications
injections, bruising from, 50
weight gain from, 34

Insulin pens, 50

Insulin pumps, 28, 75

Internet
sexual product scams, 133
websites, 121, 183–187

Intimacy, 1–6
aging and, 146–147, 152
blood glucose levels and, 73–75
emotional, 2–3, 5–6
enhancing, 89–110
by abstaining, 92–93
aphrodisiacs. *See* Aphrodisiacs
aromatherapy, 94–96
erotic media, 59, 92, 105
exercise, shared, 96–99
herbal supplements, 106–110
kissing, 91
massage, 93–96
music, 105–106
new positions/locations, 91
scents, 103–105
senses, stimulating, 103–106
sensual touching, 90–91
sexual secrets, sharing, 92
surprise, 91
time spent together, 110
scheduling, 25
without intercourse, 78, 146–147

Intrauterine devices, 86

Iyengar yoga, 22

J

Jelquing, 125

Job issues. *See* Employment

Jump Start Pledges, 25–26, 122

K

Kegel exercises, 141–142
Ketones
    low carb diets and, 43
    personal hygiene and, 50
Kissing, 91

L

Lactobacillus organisms, 84
L-arginine, 107
L-carnitine, 108
LDL cholesterol, 48–49
Levitra, 58–59, 185–186
Libido
    antidepressants and, 76
    aphrodisiacs. *See* Aphrodisiacs
    discussing with doctor, 155
    drop in, 30, 75–76
    factors affecting, 30
    herbal supplements for, 107–110
    supplement scams, 130
    testosterone and, 56, 75
Libidus, 125
Licorice, 101, 126
Lipid levels, 48–49
Lovox, 76
Low carbohydrate diets, 43, 77
Lubricants, water-based, 79

M

Maca, 109
Magic Pencil technique, 119–122

Marriage
    depression and, 17
    diabetes and, 151
    guilt and, 15
Massage, 93–96
Masturbation, 80, 81, 145
Meal planning, 148
    aphrodisiac foods, 100–102
        See also Recipes
    carbohydrate counting, 36–37
    cholesterol, dietary, 48, 49
    eating out, 36, 38, 74
    nutrition facts labels, 37
    the plate method, 35–36
    portion estimation, 36, 38
    sweating, foods that trigger, 82
    for weight loss. *See* Weight loss
Medical identification, 29
Meditation, 22, 24
Menopause
    blood glucose levels and, 74
    symptoms of, 137–138
    vaginal pain, 142–143
Men's issues
    aging, symptoms of, 138.
        See also Aging
    erectile dysfunction (ED).
        See Erectile dysfunction (ED)
    orgasm, 5
    penis enlargement scams, 125–128
    penis size concerns, 127–128
    quiz, sexual complications, 8–9
    scents, sexual arousal and, 103–104
    sexual stimulation, physical
        response to, 5
    supplement scams, 125
    weight training, 145–146
Menstruation, 74

Metformin, 41, 150

Mindfulness meditation, 24

Mixed incontinence, 141

M & M candies myths, 131

Muira puama, 109

Music
romantic, 105–106
for stress relief, 24

Mustard, 101, 172

N

Nasutra, 125

National Diabetes Information
Clearinghouse, 185

National Weight Control Registry
(NWCR), 40

Neophase, 125

Nephropathy, 23

Nerve damage. *See* Neuropathy

Nettle extract, 127

Neuropathy, 44
autonomic, 23
exercise and, 23
overflow incontinence and, 141
peripheral, 23
sweating and, 82

Nitrates, 58–59, 144

Nitroglycerin, 144

Norepinephrine, 3–4

Norplant System, 86

Nutrition facts labels, 37

O

Oats, 109

Oils
aromatherapy, 94–96
for dry skin, 83

Olive oil, 164, 167, 169, 173, 176

Olives, 101

Oral contraceptives, 86

Orgasm, 5, 80–81

Overactive bladder, 141

Overflow incontinence, 141

Oysters, 102

P

Panax ginseng, 109

Parsley, 101, 167, 169

Paxil, 76

Pedometers, 98–99

Penile implants, 66–68

Penile injections, 60–61

Penile support sleeves, 65–66

Penile suppositories, 61–62

Penile weights, 125

Penis enlargement scams, 125–128

Perimenopause symptoms, 137–138

Peripheral neuropathy, 23

Personal sexual gratification.
See Masturbation

Phenyethylamine (PEA), 3–4

Physical activity. *See* Exercise

Physical intimacy. *See* Intimacy

Physical responses
  to depression, 18
  to falling in love, 3–5
  to sexual stimulation, 5

Pillow talk, 118

Pine nuts, 101

Plate method, meal planning, 35–36

Pregnancy, fear of, 85–87

Prescription assistance programs, 31, 190–193

Problem solving, 150

Prostate problems, overflow incontinence and, 141

Prozac, 76

Public Health Foundation, 121

Q

Quiet time, 25

Quizzes, sexual complications, 8–11

R

Raspberries, 102, 168, 172

Reading, for stress relief, 25

Recipes, 103, 163–179
  appetizers/beverages:
      Chicken Drumsticks, 164
      Chocolate Almond Coffee, 165
  breads:
      Banana Ginger Muffins, 175
      Garlic Bread, 176
  breakfast/brunch:
      Chilled Melon and Berry Nectar, 166
      Fresh Herb Omelet, 167
      Yogurt with Peach Puree and Fresh Raspberries, 168
  desserts: Linda's Chocolate Log, 179
  dips/sauces/condiments:
      Guacamole, 169
      Nuom Chuc Sauce, 170
  entrees:
      Chicken Satay, 171
      Marinated Lamb Chops, 172
  soups:
      Carrot and Ginger Soup, 173
      Tortellini Soup, 174
  vegetables:
      Asparagus Soufflé, 177
      Collard Greens, 178

Rejection, fear of, 28–29

Relaxation techniques. *See* Stress

Remeron, 76

Resources, 181–187
  DVDs, 121, 182
  publications, 182–183
  websites, 183–187

Retinopathy, 23

R-rated films, 92

S

Saturated fats, 49

Saw palmetto extract, 126

Scams. *See* Sexual product scams

Scents, 103–105. *See also* Aromatherapy

Secrets
  communication and, 114
  diabetes, hiding from partners, 28
  sexual, sharing, 92

Sensual touching, 90–91

Serzone, 76

Sexual desire. *See* Libido

Sexual positions, 91

Sexual product scams, 123–133
  avoiding, 132
  breast enhancers, 128–129
  FDA's role, 132–133
  FDA warnings, 125
  libido enhancers, 130
  penis enlargement, 125–128
  reporting, 133, 185

Skin problems, 82–83

Sleep, 78
  aging and, 139–140
  interrupted, 140, 141

Spermicidal jelly, 85

Spirituality, depression and, 20

SSRI antidepressants, 76

Strawberries, 102

Stress, 20–26
  activities, eliminating, 21–22
  counseling for, 26
  friendships and, 24
  job duties, adjusting, 21
  Jump Start Pledges, 25–26
  massage and, 94
  meditation and, 22, 24
  music and, 24
  pampering and, 25
  quiet time and, 25
  sensual touching and, 90–91

Stress incontinence, 141

Sulfonylureas, 41

Sweating, excessive, 50, 82

Symlin, 41, 75

T

Teeth, caring for, 139

Testosterone, 55–58
  gels, 56, 57
  injections, 57
  low levels of
    erectile dysfunction, 55–56
    risk factors, 58
    symptoms, 56
    treatments, 56–57
  oral (buccal) tablets, 57
  patches, 57
  for women, 75

Transcendental meditation, 24

Trans fats, 49

Tribulus terrestris extract, 126

Triglycerides, 48–49

Truffles, 101

Type 2 diabetes, 14

U

U.S. Federal Trade Commission (FTC), 129, 133

U.S. Food and Drug Administration (FDA), 125, 132–133

U.S. Pharmacopeia (USP), 106

Urge incontinence, 141

Urinary incontinence, 140–142

Urinary tract infections, 83–85, 141

V

Vacuum pumps
  for breast enhancement, 128

for ED, 64–65
for penis enlargement, 125
Vagifem, 143
Vaginal area
keeping clean, 84
lubrication, 79–80, 142–143
pain, 142–143, 156
perfumes, avoiding, 84
Viagra, 58–59
ED medications and, 144
OTC versions of, 130
website address, 187
for women, 75
Vigor-25, 125
Visual stimulation, 105

W

Walking, 98–99
Water intake, 43, 82, 84
Websites, 121, 183–187
Weight gain, 34
diabetes medications and, 34, 41
hypoglycemia and, 42
insulin and, 34
testosterone and, 56
Weight loss, 34–40
calories, limiting severely, 77
carbohydrate counting, 36–37
de-emphasizing weight, 44
exercise and, 43–44
fatigue and, 77
fiber, 38–39
hypoglycemia treatment and, 42
low carbohydrate diets, 43, 77
maintenance of, 40
medications and, 41

penis size concerns and, 128
the plate method, 35–36
portion estimations, 36, 38
skipping meals, 77
tension from, 27
water intake, 43
Weight training, 145–146
Wellbutrin SR, 76
Widower's syndrome, 144
Wine, 101, 166, 170, 172, 174
Wine vinegar, 164, 170
Wolfberry, 110
Women's issues, 71–87
aging, symptoms of, 137–138.
See also Aging
antidepressants, 76
birth control, 85
bladder infections, 83–85
blood glucose levels, 73–75
alcohol, limiting, 74
exercise and, 75
menopause and, 74
menstruation and, 74
monitoring, 73–74
breast augmentation, 129–130, 183
breast enhancement scams, 128–129
communicating desires, 81.
See also Communication
diabetes medications, changing, 75
emotional responses, 116–117
estrogen supplementation, 80, 143
fatigue, 76–79
foreplay, 80, 81
herbal supplements, 107–109
hormone treatments, 75, 80, 143
household help, hiring, 78–79
libido, low, 75–76
masturbation, 80, 81

orgasm, 5, 72, 80–81
pregnancy, fear of, 85–87
quiz, sexual complications, 10–11
scents, sexual arousal and, 104–105
sexual stimulation, physical
   response to, 5
skin problems, 82–83
sweating, excessive, 82
testosterone treatment, 75
urinary tract infections, 83–85
vaginal lubrication, 79–80, 142–143
vaginal pain, 142–143, 156
yeast infections, 83–85

Y

Yeast infections, 83–85
Yoga, 22, 187
Yohimbe, 108–109

Z

Zimaxx, 125
Zoloft, 76

Other Titles Available
from the American Diabetes Association

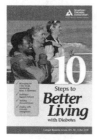

10 Steps to Better Living with Diabetes
by Ginger Kanzer-Lewis, RN, BC, EdM, CDE
Don't let diabetes take control of your life. Instead, take control of your diabetes! Learn the answers to all of your questions about self-care, including the questions you didn't even know to ask. Start living a better life with diabetes—let Ginger Kanzer-Lewis show you how.
Order no. 4882-01; Price $16.95

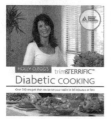

The Diabetes Dictionary
by American Diabetes Association
To stay healthy, you need to understand the constantly growing vocabulary of diabetes research and treatment. This gives you the straightforward definitions of diabetes terms and concepts you need. With more than 500 entries, this affordable, pocket-size book is an indispensable resource for every person with diabetes.
Order no. 5020-01; Price $5.95

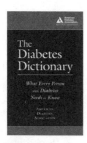

Holly Clegg's Trim & Terrific™ Diabetic Cooking
by Holly Clegg
Cookbook author Holly Clegg has teamed up with the American Diabetes Association to create a Trim & Terrific™ cookbook perfect for people with diabetes. With over 250 recipes, this collection is packed with meals that are quick, easy, and delicious. Forget the hassles of meal planning and rediscover the joys of great food!
Order no. 4883-01; Price $18.95

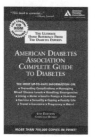

American Diabetes Association Complete Guide to Diabetes, 4th Edition
by American Diabetes Association
Have all the information on diabetes that you need close at hand. The world's largest collection of diabetes self-care tips, techniques, and tricks for solving diabetes-related problems is back in its fourth edition, and it's bigger and better than ever before.
Order no. 4809-04; Price $29.95

To order these and other great American Diabetes Association titles,
call 1-800-232-6733 or visit http://store.diabetes.org.
American Diabetes Association titles are also available in bookstores nationwide.

About the American Diabetes Association

The American Diabetes Association is the nation's leading voluntary health organization supporting diabetes research, information, and advocacy. Its mission is to prevent and cure diabetes and to improve the lives of all people affected by diabetes. The American Diabetes Association is the leading publisher of comprehensive diabetes information. Its huge library of practical and authoritative books for people with diabetes covers every aspect of self-care—cooking and nutrition, fitness, weight control, medications, complications, emotional issues, and general self-care.

To order American Diabetes Association books: Call 1-800-232-6733 or log on to *http://store.diabetes.org*

To join the American Diabetes Association: Call 1-800-806-7801 or log on to *www.diabetes.org/membership*

For more information about diabetes or ADA programs and services: Call 1-800-342-2383. E-mail: AskADA@diabetes.org or log on to *www.diabetes.org*

To locate an ADA/NCQA Recognized Provider of quality diabetes care in your area: *www.ncqa.org/dprp*

To find an ADA Recognized Education Program in your area: Call 1-800-342-2383. *www.diabetes.org/for-health-professionals-and-scientists/recognition/edrecognition.jsp*

To join the fight to increase funding for diabetes research, end discrimination, and improve insurance coverage: Call 1-800-342-2383. *www.diabetes.org/advocacy-and-legalresources/advocacy.jsp*

To find out how you can get involved with the programs in your community: Call 1-800-342-2383. See below for program Web addresses.

- *American Diabetes Month:* educational activities aimed at those diagnosed with diabetes—month of November. *www.diabetes.org/communityprograms-and-localevents/americandiabetesmonth.jsp*
- *American Diabetes Alert:* annual public awareness campaign to find the undiagnosed—held the fourth Tuesday in March. *www.diabetes.org/communityprograms-and-localevents/americandiabetesalert.jsp*
- *American Diabetes Association Latino Initiative:* diabetes awareness program targeted to the Latino community. *www.diabetes.org/communityprograms-and-localevents/latinos.jsp*
- *African American Program:* diabetes awareness program targeted to the African American community. *www.diabetes.org/communityprograms-and-localevents/africanamericans.jsp*
- *Awakening the Spirit: Pathways to Diabetes Prevention & Control:* diabetes awareness program targeted to the Native American community. *www.diabetes.org/communityprograms-and-localevents/nativeamericans.jsp*

To find out about an important research project regarding type 2 diabetes: *www.diabetes.org/diabetes-research/research-home.jsp*

To obtain information on making a planned gift or charitable bequest: Call 1-888-700-7029. *www.wpg.cc/stl/CDA/homepage/1,1006,509,00.html*

To make a donation or memorial contribution: Call 1-800-342-2383. *www.diabetes.org/support-the-cause/make-a-donation.jsp*